W9-DFY-367

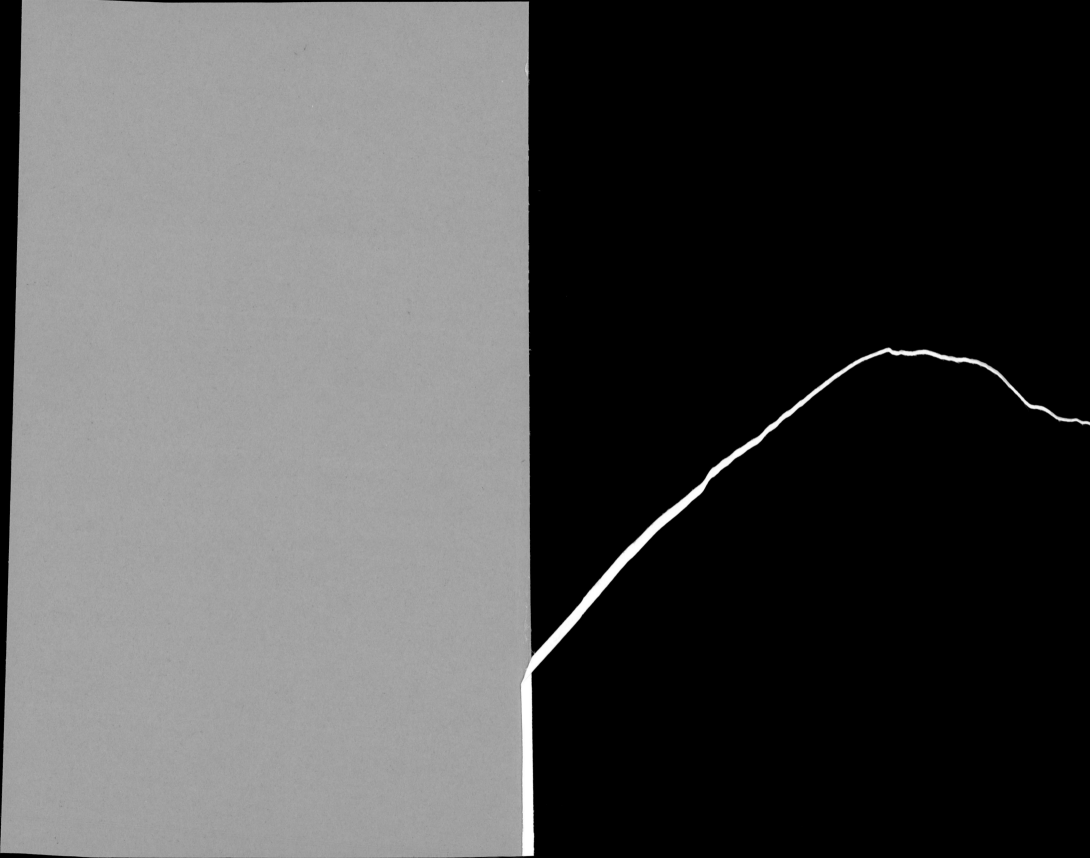

AND
THEN
WE
RISE

COMMON

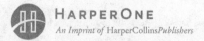

HarperOne
An Imprint of HarperCollins*Publishers*

AND
THEN
WE
RISE

A GUIDE TO LOVING AND
TAKING CARE OF SELF

The material on linked sites referenced in this book is the author's own. HarperCollins disclaims all liability that may result from the use of the material contained at those sites. All such material is supplemental and not part of the book. The author reserves the right to operate or close the website at his sole discretion following January 2024.

All scripture quotations, unless otherwise indicated, are taken from *The Holy Bible, New International Version®,* NIV® Copyright © 1973, 1978, 1984, 2011 by Biblica, Inc.® Used by permission. All rights reserved worldwide.

AND THEN WE RISE. Copyright © 2024 by Think Common Entertainment, Inc. All rights reserved. Printed in the United States of America. No part of this book may be used or reproduced in any manner whatsoever without written permission except in the case of brief quotations embodied in critical articles and reviews. For information, address HarperCollins Publishers, 195 Broadway, New York, NY 10007.

HarperCollins books may be purchased for educational, business, or sales promotional use. For information, please email the Special Markets Department at SPsales@harpercollins.com.

FIRST EDITION

Designed by Janet Evans-Scanlon
Cloud texture used throughout © korkeng/stock.adobe.com

Library of Congress Cataloging-in-Publication Data has been applied for.

ISBN 978-0-06-321517-7

23 24 25 26 27 LBC 5 4 3 2 1

All Praises and Thanks
to the MOST HIGH GOD,
Creator of the Heavens and Earth.
It is by the Grace of JESUS CHRIST
and in His Spirit I wrote this.
Thank You to All who contributed to
my path of Health and Wellness—all
the teachers, chefs, doctors, trainers,
and loved ones who supported me
on my Quest to be better.
GOD Bless You.

"Into a daybreak that's wondrously clear
I rise!"

—Maya Angelou, from "Still I Rise"

CONTENTS

INTRODUCTION

" One thought can produce millions of vibrations, and they all go back to God. "

—John Coltrane, in the album
liner notes to *A Love Supreme*

An Invitation to Elevation

Every morning, I wake up giving thanks for the day and wondering how I can be my best. I don't always feel sunny and bright, but I always know that I can find my way back there by taking certain actions. Wellness is self-love. It is a way of finding peace. It is a series of actions that connect you to your power.

There was a time in my life when I never thought about what it meant to truly love myself. The idea of taking care of myself wasn't even in my consciousness. Once I discovered that I had some say in how my day went, in how my life went, everything changed for the better. Soon into my journey of self-care, I would hit these moments when I felt like I was flying. For a while, I wondered when I was going to come back down. All these years later, I'm still soaring. That's one of the things that I've really had to learn to embrace during my practice of this lifestyle—the realization that this person I've become is who I am now. I'm not going back. I'm only going forward.

Realizing the joys that have emerged from following the path of self-care is what inspired me to write *And Then We Rise*. This book is a story about self-care in action. It is a conversation about the value of honoring and fortifying yourself. It is a guide to beginning your own journey because caring for yourself will lead you to joy and glory and will give you what you need to fly, to soar, and to be your best self consistently.

I've said before that love is the most potent force in this world. The same is true for self-love because that's where it all begins. My book *Let Love Have the Last Word* was a meditation on my love for my daughter and my community, love of God, and romantic love. *And Then We Rise* is about how to bless yourself with the warmth of your own love because in order for love to have the last word, self-love must be the first word. You've got to take care of you!

My path of wellness began with my food and ultimately helped me to become more gentle and compassionate with myself, to grow as a person, and to elevate myself spiritually. When I first started removing certain things from my diet, it gave me so much strength. As I learned how to take care of my physical body, it blessed me mentally and spiritually and emotionally. That's where my discipline comes from. Each positive choice turned out to be a seed, and as those seeds bloomed, I found myself living in a flowering garden that gives back to me continually. I call it "the beautiful present." That's a place we all deserve to live in.

There are so many dimensions to care of self. It is a physical practice and a mental practice, a soul practice and a community practice. These practices have supported me for so many years, and they were what I leaned on during the pandemic, when taking care of myself was my way of approaching all that was going on: the confusion, the chaos, the hatred, the fear. *We need to take care of ourselves. We need to take that back into the community.* It was a philosophy of love and respect that became a mantra for me.

There was a moment in my life when I realized I wanted to do something to better this world. If you want to be a part of a revolution, you've got to find those ways to be in tune with yourself. I've said it in my speeches, and I'll say it here: "There is no activism without self-activism." As Angela Davis told Afropunk, "Anyone who's interested in making change in the world also has to learn to take of herself, himself, theirself."

For Black women and Black men in America, self-care is a revolutionary act. The most fruitful and impactful human beings have had to have a certain love for self and taking care of self in order to go out and do the work they did. Those that forgot about it or strayed off that path got depleted at times. We all feel that. If you want to keep going, you've got to re-up. When you're working against dark forces, you've got to prepare yourself so that you can step forward with everything you've got.

This means blessing yourself with food that comes from the earth. Honoring yourself with a good workout. Making space for music and books and art. Embracing forgiveness and compassion. Seeking your higher self. These actions carry tremendous power. As Audre Lorde said, "Caring for myself is not self-indulgence, it is self-preservation, and that is an act of political warfare."

Take care of myself. Take care of my people. That's my way of fighting. That's my revolution.

When You Get, Give

The title *And Then We Rise* was proudly influenced by the Maya Angelou poem "Still I Rise"—my favorite poem by one of my favorite writers, ever since I was in the fifth grade. I also opened this book with some lines from that poem, because I have always revered her. As a young man, I also loved Langston Hughes, Nikki Giovanni,

Richard Wright, Ralph Ellison, James Baldwin, and Edgar Allan Poe. When I encountered the words of Dr. Angelou, I just reacted to them immediately. Her message was so clear and potent for me.

I never thought I'd get to meet her.

A time arose when I was supposed to do an event for the Common Ground Foundation, an organization we started to empower kids to become the leaders they were meant to be. Because of my filming schedule, I wasn't going to be able to fulfill that commitment, but we needed someone there to head the event.

My mother, Dr. Mahalia Hines, works with the foundation. She said, "I'm going to see if Maya Angelou can do it."

My mother didn't know Dr. Angelou, but she was able to get into contact with her and introduce her to the work our foundation was doing for the youth of Chicago. Dr. Angelou didn't know much about Common, but her great-grandson had told her enough about me that she said, "I'll be open to doing it. Let me meet the young man."

I went over to her beautiful art-filled home in Harlem. We sat in her kitchen and talked for hours, and I got to know her, and she got to know me, and she decided to do the benefit. The people were so thankful that they went from having Common to having the legendary Dr. Angelou at their event because that was a win. From that point on, we began to find ways that we could collaborate. Having the opportunity to work alongside her was monumental for me.

On one occasion, she was giving a speech at the Riverside Church, and I spoke some words to open it up. I tried to do that spontaneous talk where you speak from the heart. Then Dr. Angelou lit the spot up.

Afterwards, my aunt and some of my team were like, "Good

job." Not my mother. When I got in the car, she said, "That was not good. You could do better."

I said, "But I'm not a speaker like that."

She said, "You could be a good speaker—but you've got to work at it."

That moment changed me. My mother has been a teacher her whole life, and she knows how to tell me the truth. Because of her advice, I started to work on my speeches, and I did get better. We can only get better if we acknowledge that there is room to grow, and if we work at it. We all need teachers who can show us the path to our own greatness. You can't become better if you're convinced you're already great.

My mother is one of my teachers and mentors. So is my uncle, who was quick to teach me that if I wanted to play basketball well, I had to apply myself and do the work. So is Dr. Angelou, who touched me with her wisdom and the example she set, and who reached into the hearts of so many who learned from her writing and teachings.

I am continually moved by the efforts of some individuals to inspire and sustain others through their own example, through their leadership, and through their art. Anyone who knows me knows how much I revere John Coltrane and how much I have been influenced by his music. His album *A Love Supreme,* recorded before I was born, emerged from a spiritual quest, and that comes through to me every time I listen to it, bringing me peace and letting me sit and reflect. The sound of it can calm me, sending me into my imagination, helping me to just relax. Sometimes it sets a tone, like when I've got people around.

The album is organized into four parts: "Acknowledgement," "Resolution," "Pursuance," and "Psalm." That's something that I meditate on because it creates a beautiful framework for our own journeys through this life. Acknowledgment is the awareness and acceptance of where you are. Resolution sets you on the path. Pursuance keeps you moving in that direction. Psalm is the promised land, the place you get to inhabit if you have the commitment to keep following the dream.

What Coltrane was inspired to create through his own spiritual journey has affected so many others' journeys, including mine. When a piece of music, art, or writing touches you, it has the magical feeling of creating an energetic human relationship that exists outside of time and space. It always amazes me how people who have never met one another can be so connected, like we are part of a shared conversation, whispering the beautiful secrets of life, one to the next.

Dr. Angelou has said that she used to think she was a writer who could teach, but then she learned that she was a teacher who could write. "When you get, give," Dr. Angelou's mother taught her. "And when you learn, teach." The sharing of wisdom is a great legacy, and that's a big theme in this book.

Gifts of Healing

My journey to becoming well relates to my influences throughout my life, to the ideas I was exposed to, to the teachers I was introduced to.

As a teenager, it began with the music I was listening to.

In my twenties, it was the people I was meeting, the books I was reading, and the new way that I started eating.

In my thirties, I got into working out. I've always had a love of basketball, but actively training illuminated the connection between body, mind, and spirit.

I've spent my forties working with a wonderful therapist, and what I am learning about myself in that space sharpens my perceptions and helps me to understand who I am as a man.

Throughout my life, ever since I was a child, I have been developing my relationship with God because for me, it all comes back to the soul. I want to be my greatest self, my higher self, who can approach the world with compassion and a sense of being grounded in who I truly am.

That's why *And Then We Rise* has four parts, "The Food," "The Body," "The Mind," and "The Soul." When it comes to self-care, they are interrelated. One influences the next. My physician and I talk about mental resilience and spirituality along with physical health. My chef teaches me about how food influences how I feel mentally as well as physically. When I'm with my therapist, the conversation includes food, fitness, and faith. My pastor and I talk about mental health along with ideas of the spirit. They are all my teachers, and you'll be meeting each of them and encountering their wisdom as you read this book:

- Dr. Tracey Rico, trained in Western medicine and in holistic practices, empowers me to ask questions and know myself as part of her guidance. She's been my doctor and my teacher for a long time, and she's also worked with my mother, helping her understand the importance of food in healing. I trust her completely.

- Chef Lauren Von Der Pool is an artist, a healer, and a motivator who cooks the most delicious vegan food. She comes from the hood in DC, and she's all about helping people, helping Black women and Black men, discover the health and wellness that follows nutritional excellence. Green is life. She brings that energy to the food she makes, and she's bringing that energy to this book.

- Trainer and life coach Yancy Berry, who has been training me for a number of years, knows how to elevate me and when to push me. Yancy has knowledge, energy, awareness, and commitment, and he's going to share his thoughts on how you can create your own dedication around love of self to set goals and stick with them to take care of your body.

- Susan Shilling, my therapist, has been working with me for more than ten years. Through conversation she has illuminated my understanding of myself. A social worker who is driven by wanting to help and support people, she learned during her training that in order to help others, you have to do the work to take care of your own well-being. That's something we'll be talking about in this book. Her perspective shines a light for me, and she's here to shine a light for you, too.

- Pastor Touré Roberts always speaks from the heart and makes me feel uplifted. He comes from a spiritual place; he believes in the people in the community; and his guidance comes with practical inspiration that you can really use. I have learned so much from him and feel so connected to him, and he's been gracious enough to preach some of his ideas in this book for us.

Along my journey, I have always been compelled by this idea of living life as a continual student, always seeking knowledge. No matter how much I learn, I still feel that way, aware of how much learning there is yet to do. I didn't always have access to the kind of information that is in this book. I didn't always have the resources to do things like hire a personal chef or a trainer. That was my inspiration for putting this guide together: to gather in one place all this wisdom that I've been fortunate enough to be inspired by and grow from so I can share it here, now, with you.

And Then We Rise is about my journey, and I hope that it will be the beginning of yours. It is a call to action—because I have seen the value of nurturing yourself, taking care of yourself, building yourself up, and reinforcing your own foundations. It's about how to take all the beautiful energy that you're always offering to other people and focusing it on lighting yourself up. About taking one positive thought—you can take care of yourself—and turning it into a lifetime of positive vibrations.

You are beautiful and you are blessed, and you are worthy of your own attention, compassion, and respect, every single day.

PART 1

THE

FOOD

" It's in our lesson,
for him to know himself
To me the greatest wealth
is the best of health. **"**

—Brand Nubian, "Love vs. Hate"

From the Mic to the Speakers

I wasn't always a person who drank green juice or thought about food as a pathway to elevation. Totally the opposite! Back in the day, as a young man in Chicago, I loved French fries, fried chicken—really, anything fried and good that I could get my hands on. And don't get me started on how often I ran to Harold's Chicken Shack, Popeyes Chicken, Leon's Barbeque, Rossi's Pizza . . . I loved pork chops. I loved bacon. I loved gyros.

My mother makes incredible soul food, and that was always one of my favorite cuisines. My family would always get together, whether it was after church or during a family reunion or just on a simple day, and build love around food. My mother's cooking was her way of showing love. In the mornings, she made these amazing pancakes. My cousin, Ajile, who stayed overnight often, would always ask for her pancakes. Everybody always wanted those pancakes.

I've always had an association with food as a part of life. Food was a big loving thing for us, but healthy food was not in the conversation. I was just out there having fun with my friends, thinking about anything but my health. I was young, and I didn't know better. I hadn't made the connection between heavy food and a heavy spirit. It's all about what we have been exposed to. I can't think of one vegetarian that was in my life in those days. None of my teachers, none of my mother's friends. I didn't even know what being a vegetarian was.

My earliest introduction to that kind of consciousness came through music. One of the first records I heard as a child was *The Message* by Grandmaster Flash and the Furious Five, back in 1982. I was only ten years old. I still remember thinking about that album and about whether or not I should buy it. The title song was such a conscious rap, and I listened closely to Melle Mel rapping about awareness of the environment we were living in and how it affected our health. "It's like a jungle sometimes / It makes me wonder how I keep from goin' under," and "Can't stop to turn around, broke my sacroiliac / A mid-range migraine, cancered membrane." When I listened to it, it got to me.

I was sixteen when KRS-One put out "My Philosophy." He was rapping about being artists, scholars, and teachers. You could hear the pride in that song. He wasn't there to "reinforce stereotypes of today / Like all my brothers eat chicken and watermelon / Talk broken English and drug selling." He sang about walking around with heads high, being really clear about what he was about, calling himself "an intelligent brown man / A vegetarian, no goat or ham / Or chicken or turkey or hamburger / Cause to me that's suicide, self-murder."

Through listening, I was learning from KRS how the foods we eat affect us. Those lyrics made me understand what being a vegetarian is about.

I began rapping those lyrics with conviction, rapping the lyrics as if I was an expert, even though I wasn't there yet. I wasn't even fully processing what he was saying, but the more I said it, the stronger I felt. I wasn't a vegetarian—I might even have been eating chicken while I was saying it! But it's that exposure. That song was like a musical mantra for me at sixteen because it was reaffirming and introducing me to the idea of loving myself. I felt like he was encouraging me to be my greatest self and to be proud of who I am.

Then there was Eric B. & Rakim. In "Paid in Full," Rakim raps "Me and Eric B. and a nice big plate of / Fish, which is my favorite dish / But without no money, it's still a wish." They were talking about eating healthier in their raps, and it was cool and it was empowering.

Rapping what KRS-One and Rakim were saying just made me feel good as a Black man, and made me feel strong as a Black man. So did Brand Nubian, whose song "Wake Up" says plainly, "The solution knowledge of self to better ourself / 'Cause I know myself, that we can live much better than this," feeding us wisdom that revolved around self-awareness and self-love.

That's what a lot of hip hop brought to us. Specifically, KRS-One, Brockhampton, Big Daddy Kane, Brand Nubian, and A Tribe Called Quest had those lyrics that made me say, "Oh, man, I love being me."

That was great mental food. People think of rap as being aggressive, talking about the tough parts of the street—the hustle that goes on in the street—and partying. When I first experienced hip hop, some of the music was just fun and some had that consciousness to it. Much of it was about love for self and love for your community and being there to take care of others for real.

Brand Nubian was another iconic group who inspired me with their wisdom, though I didn't truly know how salient the lyrics were at that time: "It's in our lesson, for him to know himself / To me the greatest wealth is the best of health." Today, those words hit differently. Powerfully.

Hip hop planted the seeds for my change. It didn't fully emerge at that young age, but it was there, waiting for more exposures to really grow and take root within me.

Like KRS said, "The lecture is conducted from the mic into the speaker."

The words came first. The conviction came later.

Food Is Love

I believe in the healing aspects of food. Some foods give you energy. Some take that energy away from you. We've all experienced the way food affects us. You drink alcohol, you feel it in your body. You drink coffee, you feel it. You drink a green juice every morning, you feel that, too. What we put in our bodies has an impact, for better or for worse. When I'm filming, when I have to perform, I'm even more conscious of what I'm putting in my body because when I'm in a creative space, I need to feel it in my gut. Heavy foods take that away from me.

If you came over to my house in the morning, I might offer you a glass of green juice or a superpowered smoothie. If it were dinnertime, I might offer you a plate of broccoli, cauliflower, mushrooms, and tofu. This kind of food makes me feel like a higher version of myself and sets me up right to do all the things I want to spend my time doing. That's why I drink those green drinks; that's my coffee. Early in my career, I used to get sick often and experience a lot of congestion, but in my thirties, when I removed dairy from my diet, I started noticing how clear I sounded vocally. When you see the difference, when you feel the difference, that's when it stays with you. That's been my path: not just doing something because someone else says that it's right, but learning from exposure, making a change, and feeling the impact.

One of the people in my life to whom I am always turning for information about my health, Dr. Tracey Rico, is an integrative medicine specialist. She worked in an emergency room for thirty years, and she's also trained in holistic practices, so I really trust her when it comes to how I take care of my body. She believes in evidence, and she believes in the connection between mind and body. She is always empowering me to ask questions, to understand what I need to do for my body so that I can live at my most powerful every day. When we talk about health, we get into the food that people eat, how much we move around in a day, and how smoking damages the body. We also talk about why it's so important to be positive. As she says, mind is always more important than matter, and negative thoughts can harm you. If we become more positive, exercise more, lose the cigarettes, spend time hiking or in nature, we experience life in a renewed way.

That green juice is more than a beverage. It's a choice I make every day to flood my body with the best chance to power myself up for a healthier future. What I've learned from Dr. Tracey is that sickness is not jumping out at you from the dark randomly for the most part. Chronic illness—heart disease, diabetes, high blood pressure—is an accumulation of choices over time.

Having a donut for breakfast every morning instead of fruit isn't neutral. It sets off a chain of events in the body. Over a year, over ten years, over twenty, the impact of that choice gets bigger and bigger. Dr. Tracey has told me again and again that illness is not guaranteed. If your health is a result of your choices, then what choices can you make right here, right now, today, to support your lifelong strength and vitality? As you get started on our journey of self-care, here's something to keep in mind: What are the little things that you're choosing every day? These small, barely acknowledged actions add up. If you can shift a repetitive practice, like what you eat and drink in the morning every single day, that equals growth. Over the years, that single daily action represents thousands of opportunities for healing and repair.

It seems intuitive when you think about a car. A car needs oil and gas. If you put sugar or water in a gas tank, you're not going to get far. We need to think about that when it comes to what we put in our bodies, too. You might grab that cup of coffee for that immediate rush of energy because in those moments, you're not thinking about five years from now. You're just trying to make it through the day, through this next thing you need to do.

If you're just focused on getting through the next hour, a coffee and donut will do it because you get the sugar, you get the caffeine, to keep moving.

Over a lifetime, you're going to need a different kind of energy to keep you going.

The Acknowledgment

When I was nineteen, I was in Los Angeles for the first time. I was with No I.D. and Twilite Tone, two of my closest friends. These are guys I started out with, who produced my first album, and we were in LA promoting *Can I Borrow a Dollar?*

It was a sunny day in October, and we had just eaten in a diner on Sunset, a place that had become like our second home. I ordered my regular breakfast: pork chop and eggs, toast, orange juice. I was enjoying that pork when No I.D. said, "Man, Rash"—as you know, my real name is Rashid—"when are you going to start taking care of yourself? When you going to start thinking about yourself?"

Me and No I.D. and Twilite Tone had all come from the South Side of Chicago, eating and living in a way that our culture culti-vated and taught us. Where we grew up, the Nation of Islam was all around us. Members of the Nation were dressed in their suits, preaching about fasting and morality, spirituality and loyalty. What I most remember was just how much they believed that being healthy was actually holy. My friends, through their connection to the Nation, started practicing discipline and knowledge of self and giving up food like pork. What they didn't know was that I had been learning about the Nation, too, about those ideas of love of self, and that eating well could be a spiritual practice and a beautiful thing.

No I.D. was an intelligent guy and a very persuasive guy, always trying to convince you to do as much right as possible. From a very young age, he had a focus about him, and it always seemed like he had become a man before we did.

Still, I felt this inner resistance. I think I laughed. I was saying to myself, *Well, I'm going to keep eating pork*, and thinking, *I'm not going to listen just because y'all think y'all know something that I don't.*

Even with that resistance within me, I could see a glimpse of light coming from them, as if these brothers were shining because they were practicing this discipline. We all want to shine like that.

Maybe that's why something clicked with me as we left the diner. I remember it clearly, just walking across the street with the blue skies above me on that beautiful sunny day. It was like a mirror was put in front of me, as if I was watching myself resisting and being ignorant. There's a point in life where no matter how we were raised, each individual starts to see what resonates with them, asking themselves, *Who am I, and what things do I really want for myself?* With those questions before me, my resistance flowed away.

It was still a new thing for me to make it active. All those foods were a part of my culture—barbecue ribs, pork chops, ham sandwiches, bacon. Things I really enjoyed. I was thinking, *I want to see how this is going to work. Can I do this?*

Before that point, it felt easier to stay in the space of what I was used to. I had the attitude that so many of us have, where what we are doing is just what we do. As if this is the way we grew up, this is where we're going to remain, and other people urging us towards change actually makes us shut down. That feeling that no matter what anybody says, you are just not going to change. I had been resisting for that reason. But as I looked in that mirror, as I watched that scene play out, I knew there was something deeper happening and I wanted better for myself. I realized that I deserved better and that I was going to strive for better. It was one of the first times where I started to really think for myself and think about loving myself in that way. This was a moment of change for me. By the time I crossed that street, I had decided to take pork out of my diet.

From that moment, my awareness around food started to grow. For instance, it was the custom for me and my friends to close our evenings out with a late-night stop for food at a place we called the Dirty Burger. It was open until four in the morning, so we'd go there after drinking for pizza puffs, gyros, cheeseburgers, French fries, all of it. That was just the way of life.

I remember being at the Dirty Burger one night, and when I got home, I was just not feeling well. The food tasted good, but I didn't feel good. I decided to stop eating beef for a week or two. As a result, my sleep was better. I was waking up feeling lighter. After two weeks, I ate beef again, and the next morning, I just felt so heavy in my body, and it wasn't the way I wanted to feel. That's when I said to myself, "I don't need any more research. I know what I need to do."

I moved from eating beef burgers to eating turkey burgers; I found a grocery store that carried turkey burgers so I could have them at home. I stayed in that space for a while. My body told me what I needed, and what I needed was to feel light, to sleep well.

In those early days of not eating pork, not eating beef, I felt like I was doing something for myself. It was a period of unlearning some of the things that had been passed down for survival by the generations before me. Acknowledging that some of those things might not be beneficial for me at this time in my life. Sometimes we think it's easier not to change, but things actually get easier when we do the hard thing of change because life becomes so much softer once you've persevered through it.

The thing to remember as you discover your own changes is that the benefits you feel will be personal to you, and they don't always happen overnight. It can be weeks and months of trying something new to see what the effects will be once it takes hold. It does take time, but you will feel it.

The Resolution

I moved from Chicago to New York when I was twenty-six, and Brooklyn became my home, a place of new adventure. I was hanging around with some people who were eating vegetarian in a way that was just really down-to-earth and also totally about elevation. Just being in that environment and having exposure to a community that was mostly vegan and into the arts and bettering themselves had an impact on me. We'd go out to juice bars, and when I drank those juices, when I ate that food, I experienced a rebirth in many ways.

My father used to always tell me to drink carrot juice and aloe vera. Discovering it for myself within my peer group, however, was a whole other level. I was changing the relationship I had with my food and developing a deeper understanding of how food made my body feel, and it was all connected to my creative and spiritual journey. Eating plants, creating this energy in my days, was giving me a new energy around understanding how my choices affect me in all areas. I saw that I had control over myself to not eat certain addictive foods, and that I could improve my health and quality of life through simple practices like getting more sleep and eating more greens. Over time, I started working on my physical health through training, and I was working out harder than I'd ever worked out before. I began meditating and praying every morning. It felt natural.

As a musician, I was starting new projects at the same time that I was developing this new clarity and having more energy. I was being more open, and in my seeking I was finding and discovering things on a higher vibration. Through music, I found things within myself that I didn't know I had. It felt like I was becoming a new person. Sixteen-year-old me got me to this moment with my heart, by putting my heart into things and being really true to my heart, taking the time to understand what my heart felt and not being afraid to express that or expose it and share it. That's really how I got here. I don't think I have always given myself the credit that the younger me deserves for being willing to do that. For having the courage to leave something behind and be present with the future ahead of me.

When I first released my music, within the industry, things were really thriving, and people were starting to have big records and commercial success, and hip hop was sprouting out. I had a lot of learning to do about who I wanted to become, but I knew who I was. And I expressed that. I was a Chicago dude who studied at an HBCU. I have an incredible mother who was a teacher, and I also grew up around gangbanging. I grew up going to church and grew up drinking and fighting, too. I was able to bring all of that to who I was and not try to be something else. I was going to New York but not trying to be New York, and I wasn't trying to be LA, even though those are both hip hop juggernaut cities, with New York being the mecca in the beginning and LA being the next place that flourished and blew up.

They both influenced me, but I still was able to be me, coming from a pure place of using my heart and love for what I do. I was proud to be talking about Chicago and saying our slang. I didn't let the pursuit of success usurp the pursuit of love and creativity and purpose and my goal of really injecting something important into my community. That was very important to me, and it still is. That love comforted me: if this one project isn't successful, I love what I do, so I'll work on the next. I didn't go where my heart didn't tell me to go because my heart has love for God, for my people, for my community, and for the art form. By putting that love into it, putting my heart into those things, it removed the sheer hype and the glitz of the pursuit, and it removed the false aspects of what I could have done to pursue this. With the love, you can work on the heart as you do it.

What's gotten sixteen-year-old Rashid to where I am now is that when I find something I love, I go for it. Whether working through difficult situations or working on my health or working on an artistic or athletic goal, I choose what I'm going to focus on. It starts as a choice, and it becomes a routine and what I do automatically.

As we grow up, we are exposed to new ideas, and some of them fit with who we are and who we are growing into. I didn't know about Basquiat when I was young. There were filmmakers I hadn't been exposed to. As I moved through the world, I was exposed to new things. My taste evolved, changed, and grew, but I had to have that exposure to it for that to happen. A lot of things that you experience in life come from what you were presented with, and that helps determine what you think is good. We do hope to find our own individuality and perspective on what is good for us, and we can only learn that by sampling the different things around us. It was about saying to myself: *How can I be better? What things are working well in my life, and how can I adopt this as a way of living every day?*

When I ate better, I felt better. It wasn't just an external thing. I was learning how to be present with a new clarity. By changing my ways, I was also changing my view of myself. Finding this new discipline and self-affirming routines boosted my confidence, and that type of energy started coming out like an aura around me. My work started to take on new forms. My voice started to change. It had a clarity to it. I noticed that strength and presence. That the better I ate, the more creative I became.

The Pursuance

Once I made this very positive connection between how I fed myself and how I felt, I couldn't stop. I began seeking out those people who could guide me in my search for deeper understanding about how I could take care of my physical body through the food I was eating.

Dr. Tracey believes that the ideal diet consists of eating whole foods—that is, the way you find them in nature—and eating mostly plants. It goes back to what our bodies are made of, she told me. "We're not made of Tylenol and Claritin," she said. "We're not made of preservatives." As life forms, we're made of carbohydrates, fats, protein, and vitamins and minerals, like salt, potassium, calcium, zinc, vitamin C. We're made of water.

Dr. Tracey advocates for eating a lot of plants instead of eating processed foods because factory food is designed to make money, not create health. Those factory foods are often stripped of nutrition, and all the goodness has been replaced by preservatives and chemicals that allow them to sit on a shelf for four years. Like Dr. Tracey reminds me, bread used to actually spoil, cheese used to actually spoil, milk would spoil. Fill them with preservatives so that they never spoil, and they're not real food anymore. Instead of eating food products, we need to be eating food.

What does it take to heal the body? A functioning immune

system and the resources to heal. What your blood vessels are made of is what your body needs to function, and those nutrients are in whole plants, fresh foods, green foods. If you want healthy skin, it's not about putting lotion on your skin. It's about giving yourself that good protein, those healthy fats. That's what makes the glow come through.

There is a place in Honduras run by Dr. Sebi, an herbalist known for his approach to food and the body. When I visited, we went into the hot springs, and we fasted, and we ate some of the purest and cleanest foods I've had, herbs and vegetables fresh from the land. I felt like I could just fly. It was amazing. I had a glow like I had never had before in my life.

Dr. Sebi's daughter Xave had been consulting with me, teaching me about the various herbs, and the benefits of eating a more alkaline diet, with a focus on fruits and vegetables, no processed food. When I was in Baltimore filming *Luv*, a movie about the development of a young adolescent boy who idolizes his formerly incarcerated uncle (me), I asked Xave if she knew a vegan chef in the DC area who could prepare that kind of food. She connected me with Lauren Von Der Pool, the Queen of Green, who is a bright spirit, a chef, and an artist.

When I first met Lauren, I had no idea how much I would learn from her. It's only when I look back that I can say, *Wow, that person changed my life*. She's been a big part of giving me the energy that I need in my body along with an understanding that what I eat affects how I feel. Her knowledge of food and nutrition helps me feel like I'm at my best and helps me operate at my highest levels.

She's taught me about the power of juices, protein shakes, and eating green. I want to be clear on this: you can eat vegan and still not be healthy. You can eat vegan and it's all fast food and it's all processed food and it's all fake bacon. Or you can eat the greens, the fruits, the vegetables, the seeds, the protein.

Those first few days in Baltimore, I was getting deliveries of her food, but she felt that it would be something special if she could cook for me in person. They had just gotten me a new trailer and it had a stove, so Lauren came in her chef gear. Her energy and her spirit made me feel so good and charged, inspired and happy. Before I saw her cooking, I didn't even know that this much love was being put in the meal, but when I got the full experience, I could feel from her that she loved what she was doing, that she really was aware of what she was doing, and that she cared for my well-being. She didn't know me well, but she just cared.

That was the moment that I said, "Can you come and cook every day?"

She just brought so much life. Everyone on the shoot, even people who weren't vegan, started coming to my trailer to eat lunch. That's how much they were digging her foods. Even people that had no desire to eat vegan were like, *This is luscious.*

Lauren can go anyplace and bring some joy to the room. Her energy is part of what makes her food so good, and that's part of her belief system around food, too. "I always believe that we impact the food as much as the food is impacting us," she said. "It's a conversation; it's a relationship. It goes back to where the food comes from, and then, who's making the food? There's energy that goes into that food. If someone has negative energy and they're cooking for you, you're also eating that frequency. It is intertwined in food." When I eat Lauren's food, I can feel that energy, I can feel that love, I can feel that frequency.

As I've gotten to know Lauren, I've learned more about the path that brought her to this space of teaching and sharing. She grew up in DC eating chicken wings with mumbo sauce and started her vegan journey at sixteen with a raw food diet. She believes that food is sacred and special, and she has done justice work around food and obesity with Michelle Obama. Cooking is a divine expression for her, and her ideas about food have touched my life and opened my eyes to this beautiful way of eating.

The food she makes is powerful in so many ways, which is why I introduced her to Venus and Serena Williams. Consider that these are two women who rely on their physical strength as professional athletes. What they eat crystalizes their performance abilities; they need a level of commitment and dedication that the average person can't even imagine. This plant-based food has touched their lives, too.

I feel blessed to get to eat the meals that she prepares. It is a rare privilege to have someone like Lauren spend her time and energy creating the kind of food that leaves you feeling energized, nourished, connected. The beautiful thing is that Lauren's philosophy is available to everyone through her books, her retreats, and her presence online. I've learned from her teaching as much as from the plates she creates, and through that, my mother has also been learning and changing the way she thinks about eating.

We all need to eat plants. You are what you consume on every level, and what you eat, you become. If you eat more plants, Lauren told me, then you're going to get more oxygen to your cells and you're going to be able to think more clearly. Your body is going to be clean and clear enough to be that vessel, to get those spiritual downloads, to get that inspiration. All of it works together. A lot of us separate ourselves and compartmentalize, but we're whole beings. Everything is connected.

Lauren has taught me that what you eat becomes a part of your entire molecular structure, which includes the brain. In that way, good food is basically medicine that is growing all around us. "The reality of life is bigger than a restaurant, bigger than a grocery store, even bigger than a farmer's market," Lauren said. "All these things are coming from our Mother Earth. Exploring and seeing what the earth is offering around you is going to make a huge difference." By just incorporating more plants into your life, she believes, you're going to feel and see a difference.

Her advice is to look for fruits and vegetables that are organically grown or wild, or that are local, because when the soil is so tampered with, the nutrition is lacking. "You can taste the difference if you travel abroad," she said. "Right overseas in the Caribbean, the difference in the flavor of the food and the fruits and vegetables is absolutely different from the flavor and the potency of the food in America because a lot of it is genetically modified and also a lot of it is grown in soil that isn't rich.

"Your food is your medicine. If you're eating a burger every day, just look at the impact it's having on your digestion. A lot of people are compounding meal on top of meal on top of meal without actually releasing anything. Your body becomes a cemetery. Your body becomes a cesspool for toxins, worms, parasites. You don't want that. You want to be able to feel good, to not hold that disease in the body. That's why the earth provides us with herbs, it's medicine. If you eat that burger, make sure that the next day you take a digestive herb, like burdock root, to make sure it doesn't stay in your system. If you're going to have alcohol, drink burdock root and dandelion root because you know that's going to flush your kidneys and your liver and help to enrich your blood.

"Have fun, but understand the possibilities that are out there for you—what you're doing, how to navigate those decisions. It allows for freedom. It allows for people to feel like they aren't in a box. It's so multilayered, talking about mental illness and relating it to food. There are some people who become so obsessed with food and trying to be perfect and healthy. We're addicted to food. We can't get enough of it. It's not to say that you can't have an indulgent moment and enjoy something; it's to understand the adverse elements and how to combat that."

What I love about Lauren's perspective is that she doesn't imagine that we are going to only eat this way, all of the time. "You can do anything you want," she said, "and have the wisdom to do what makes sense. If you want to enjoy yourself for a moment, equip yourself with the knowledge to make sure that these things don't stay in your body."

You can start by drinking more water, or start with some green. Put some greens in your meals, some vegetables. Then go to green drinking. I'm not going to suggest that if you stop drinking coffee and start drinking green drinks that you'll love it right away. You don't need to wake up tomorrow with a whole new way of doing everything. Change can take years, and that's okay. Taste is developed. Every time you do something, you're developing your taste for it.

It's okay for you to take it slow as you find what works for you. Try to prepare your food in a different style—see how it feels. Order more vegetables at the restaurant. I like Chinese food, like broccoli with tofu, eggplant, carrots, mushrooms, a side of rice, maybe some dumplings. Ethiopian food always has plenty of vegetables. Even at a pizza place, I can get a pizza with tomato sauce and vegetables. Most restaurants have something that is good that I want to eat.

I want us to eat well! Really well! I'd just like to redefine what good food really is: tasty and delicious in the moment—and good for your body, too.

The Psalm

My life is full and busy. Slowing down to eat a meal is, for me, a small measure of the divine in this world. Before I eat, I say grace and thank God for the food. I've always said grace before my meals; it started when I was really young, a family thing that my mother instilled in me. She taught me to say grace so early in my life that I can't even point you to the moment when it began because it was just what we did before every meal. That moment of gratitude, when I thank God, is such a part of me.

When my team and I went on a retreat, a break for us to breathe a little and get away from the day-to-day grind, the retreat leader talked with us about mindful eating and continuous gratitude to food. When we were asked to pause and thank the food, it felt awkward at first. That's how it is when we do something new. We have to relax and try and see how it really feels instead of leaning into that natural resistance.

"Thank you for being green," I said. I looked around and I could see the others saying their words. "Thank you for what you are going to do when I eat you."

It took a moment for me to make the connection between the grace I had been taught to say as a kid and this idea of being conscious about food, about where it comes from and how it makes me feel. I'll admit, it took me a little while to get really into it. Once I did, it made me feel so connected. When the two came together, it made perfect sense to me.

When I say grace, I'm talking directly to God, who gave us this food. This time, we added on to that. We gave thanks to the people who grew the vegetables and fruits. We gave thanks to the people who drove the trucks. We gave thanks to the people who sold it at the grocery store. With each layer, I felt more and more connected to the green vegetables, to the sweet potato, to everything that was on my plate, about to give me the energy to enjoy this day with these wonderful people. I must have said grace a million times in my lifetime, and I will continue to do so. Pausing to appreciate every individual who participated in the process that brought this meal to my plate gave me a whole new level of appreciation and thankfulness.

Gratitude is an embracing of the goodness of the people around us and the gift that God has given us in food. When we pause, we are spiritually connecting with the chain of people and created things that make our journey to well-being and self-care possible through each plate. When we take time to be grateful for the lives that we have and the things that we are eating, we sow the seed of wellness into our lives. This is a centering practice we can all learn to do, wherever we are, whenever we eat. It is honoring the stomach. It is honoring the tongue. It is honoring the gut. It is honoring the brain. It is honoring the digestive tract. It is honoring the soil, the seed, the water, the person who planted it, the person who processed it, the person who made it with goodness and grace.

Learning to honor myself with this process is part of my journey, too. When I'm on set, every time Lauren makes me a meal, she'll write down what I'm about to eat and, below it, an affirmation. I love those sticky notes, and I take them home with me, where they live on a wall in my kitchen, a collection of brightly colored reminders about the relationship between eating well and feeling well.

They say things like:

I am love.
I am fresh!
I am a blessing.
I live bravely in my true authenticity.
I am an embodiment of God's grace.

The whole process of eating is part of the language of life that is happening between our bodies, our food, and our spirits. Whenever I'm getting a glass of water or something to eat, those affirmations sing out loud to me, reminders that I am worth my own time and worthy of joy.

Food Is Community

Food is so personal for people. It's a way of showing love, of sharing what we have, of experiencing a moment with other people. But food is not just social. It's also a personal moment you have with yourself because what you eat is how you're going to feel later. It's natural to feel a pull when it comes to socializing because you just want to participate and be part of the group. It's also okay to find that path where you are taking care of your own needs and not just putting what other people want from you ahead of what you want for yourself.

Daily Doses of Health and Power

I've learned that when I'm reaching for a snack, the body is wired to go for the easiest thing available. We eat with our eyes before food ever makes it to our mouths. If the potato chips are on the counter, that's probably what you'll have. That's just nature in action. If all you see are apples, oranges, mangoes, you're more likely to eat from the fruit bowl. When you get hungry, there it is: fresh food, fast.

I'm not a cook, and I'll never pretend to be. My mom, she's the cook in the family. I'm the one who can make a smoothie. We can all do that! Lauren feels that a blender is a great tool to invest in because you can use it for juicing, for smoothies, for dressings, to make your own almond butter to put on some apples as a healthy, energizing snack. It doesn't have to be the most expensive one, just something to get the job done.

As Lauren says, juicing is so effective that it activates you immediately. According to her, it can heal you on a cellular level, detox your body, energize you. Depending on what it is you're juicing, you're going to get different effects because foods have different minerals and benefits and energetics. You can absolutely achieve so many great benefits just by throwing some fruit and vegetables into a blender.

Try:

A turmeric shot in the morning

Green juice for energy

Apples with almond butter as a snack

Nuts and seeds for protein

Eating more greens, all day

Burdock root and dandelion after drinking alcohol

A green smoothie

Chopped veggies with cilantro mustard dressing

CILANTRO MAPLE-MUSTARD NECTAR

"I can literally drink my Maple-Mustard Nectar, and I have on a few occasions! It is sweet and tangy with a twist of exotic flair from the extra-virgin coconut oil. Excellent for the skin and easy on the palate, this flavorful nectar is a total win/win!"

—Lauren

SERVES 4–6

TOOLS: Blender

INGREDIENTS

1 cup extra-virgin coconut oil

¼ cup apple cider vinegar

¼ cup grade B maple syrup

2 heaping tablespoons mustard

2 tablespoons freshly chopped cilantro

¼ of a red onion

1 tablespoon onion powder

Nama shoyu, to taste

Pink Himalayan sea salt, to taste

DIRECTIONS

1. Put the coconut oil, apple cider vinegar, maple syrup, mustard, cilantro, red onion, onion powder, nama shoyu, and salt into a blender and blend until smooth.

2. Enjoy the nectar on salad!!

SPICY MANGO CHUTNEY

"I love mangoes so much that it is only right that I put my gorgeous Spicy Mango Chutney recipe in this book. It takes less than 5 minutes to make. I use it on lots of dishes and I hope that you have just as much fun with it as I do!"

—Lauren

SERVES 4–6

TOOLS: Food processor

INGREDIENTS

½ Scotch bonnet pepper

½ cup sliced scallions

2 cups fresh organic tomatoes

3 whole mangoes, chopped

4 Medjool dates

1 teaspoon onion powder

Pink Himalayan sea salt, to taste

DIRECTIONS

1. Place the pepper and scallions into a food processor with 1 cup of tomatoes. Blend until the pepper is fully ground up.

2. Add the remaining 1 cup of tomatoes, mangoes, dates, onion powder, and salt. Pulse until desired consistency is reached.

3. Remove the chutney from the processor and enjoy!

GRAND SLAMMIN' TACOS

"My girls Serena and Venus love my Grand Slammin' Tacos. These tacos are fresh, yummy, and super easy to make! Give them a whirl, and maybe you'll be grand slammin', too!"

—Lauren

SERVES 4–6

TOOLS: Juice or food processor, dehydrator

INGREDIENTS

Nutmeat

3 cups almonds, soaked overnight

1 Vidalia onion, diced

3 cloves fresh garlic

2 jalapeños, diced and seeded

3 tablespoons extra-virgin olive oil

2 tablespoons paprika

2 tablespoons onion powder

2 tablespoons pink Himalayan sea salt

1 tablespoon cumin

1 tablespoon garlic powder

Toppings

2 tomatoes, diced

1 red onion, diced

1 avocado, diced

2 jalapeños, sliced

1 cup romaine lettuce, diced

½ cup sour cream

Taco Shells

6 red or white cabbage leaves

DIRECTIONS

1. Run the almonds through your juicer or food processor until they have a nice meaty texture.

2. Add the onion, garlic, jalapeños, olive oil, paprika, onion powder, salt, cumin, and garlic powder to the juicer or food processor, mixing them in very well.

3. Place on a Teflex sheet and throw in the dehydrator overnight.

4. The next day, add the nutmeat to your taco shells and add your desired toppings.

5. ¡Buen apetito!

When I first became a vegan, there was a Thanksgiving where the changes I was making seemed to be affecting everyone else along with me. On this particular holiday, I was eating in this new way, and because it was so fresh for me, it was startling for others to witness this change. It felt like some people who were there were frustrated with me, as if I was making waves by what I was choosing to have on my plate. The fact that I wasn't eating the food that my mother prepared for this feast was confusing to the other people at the table. All I could do was not concern myself too much with their concern about how I was changing my life for the better. They worry about you, you worry about them worrying, as if you're doing something wrong by trying to do right by yourself—it's too much.

The one person there who accepted it all with calm and grace was my mother. Cooking is my mother's way of embracing me, one of her ways of showing love, and for the next Thanksgiving, she made sure to make some vegetarian food for me. Throughout the meal, she kept asking how it was. I said that it was okay, but just okay, because the truth was, it was bland. I was grateful, but I wasn't going to lie to her.

She said, "I'm going to figure out how to make it really good."

And she did.

She still makes collard greens. She still makes candied yams; she used agave instead of sugar. My mom took that love she had, that she was putting in all of the ham or the spaghetti or the turkey, and just started putting that same love into meals that I can enjoy. She realized that she could season the meal well, and those seasonings actually make it healthier because those herbs and spices that she started adding—thyme, ginger, basil, parsley, black pepper—are more than flavor enhancers. They're what Lauren calls medicine.

On this journey to becoming vegan, when I was still eating fish, one of my favorite dishes was my mom's catfish. It's just amazing. Now I'm back to eating vegan, but that's not to say that I will never eat fish again in my life. I'm just paying attention to how I feel, what my body is asking for, what will give me that enjoyment now and also later. It's not about a rule, or doing something right or wrong.

Talking to family about making these kinds of changes can lead to some teasing or looks or even actual arguments. It's courageous to have those conversations, and it's important to acknowledge how hard these changes can be. For myself, I know that I am committed to this path, and I will still feel challenged by certain environments. Every time I go back home, I recommit myself to making positive choices. I may have changed, but Chicago is still full of all that good-tasting food that I associate with a good time. Harold's Chicken is still there, and when I see my friends eating that, I have to take a moment and remember what I really want.

When I moved to New York and experienced the support of a community practicing a vegan and healthy lifestyle around me, that helped me, but the masses don't practice it, which turns making different choices with our food into a revolution on so many levels. A lot of things that are being told to us and sold to us are counterproductive to health. They're pushed as if they are blessings, when really, it's the opposite. Advertisers are promoting alcohol, and the people in the ads look happy and healthy and like they are having a great time. Same goes for beef ads. I see those commercials every time I watch sports, and then I'm listening to the broadcasters talk about all the steaks they're eating. It's all around us, and saying no to that and yes to health can feel like we're going against the norm. If you want to think in a different way, outside of what the masses and the culture are doing, you have to find a power within yourself to do that. You have to find the reason behind it. You have to find belief behind it and find inspiration in new places. You've got to surround yourself with an environment that encourages it so that you can actually see happy people doing the things that make them healthy, so you know it's for real.

"Black Food: Liberation, Food Justice, and Stewardship" is a conversation between food justice warrior Karen Washington and Bryant Terry, food activist and author/editor of the cookbooks *Vegan Soul Kitchen* and *Black Food*. In the course of their talk, which can be accessed online at www.bioneers.org, Terry said, "It's not just about food as fuel: it's about life, it's about connection, it's about love, it's about all these things that capitalism has stripped it of."[1]

It's a challenge to unlearn what we have spent so many years learning. Advertising is one thing—we know the advertisers don't care about us. What makes it so hard is not just the advertising culture. It's our personal culture, the one that we love, that we've inherited from the generations before us. It's a comfortable place for us, and it takes a lot to step out of anything that your culture has been practicing for so long. It takes a whole lot because it's a part of your family and a part of your community. But so are so many healthy foods.

In his conversation with Washington, Terry went on to say, "I'm not denying that Black folks like to eat red velvet cake, mac 'n' cheese, and ribs, but what about collards, mustard greens, turnips, dandelion, sugar snap peas, pole beans, black-eyed peas, sweet potatoes, butternut squash, kale? These are our traditional foods. These are the types of food that have sustained our people for generations . . . We should be embracing these foods because it's our birthright. They were there before us, and they've sustained our people through the roughest times, and they can help address the exponential rise in preventable diet-related illnesses that we see in our communities."

The food you learned from your family, what you ate at home, isn't put there by your grandmother because she wants to hurt you. You know that there's love in that food. When you eat it, you taste that love, you feel that love. Yet that same food may not be loving your body, may not be making you feel strong and beautiful, even though your heart is full.

I do believe that food now is just different because we live in a different time. When my great-grandmother was eating those collards with pork, the meat was straight from Mississippi, and it wasn't full of all the hormones and additives that are regularly put in meat today. All you have to do is look at the cows and you can see it—they're stressed out. It's not the same food that our grandmothers were eating. The recipes haven't changed; the ingredients have changed; it's okay for the way we think about food to evolve accordingly.

I feel blessed that my mom was willing to prepare food in a new way. Because of her love for me, she learned how to do it. Human beings learn from one another. That's what we do. I'm learning from other people. People in my family have learned from me. My mom was all about the soul food when I was young, and she's making food in that style and with those flavors, she just has shifted her preparation in some ways to incorporate more vegetables. She learned how to do it because of her love and support for me, and now she does it because she herself wants to be healthy.

One of my favorite things is still to sit down and have a good meal with people I love. It's not like you need to never have a family meal again. I'm not asking you to give up everything about who you are. The point is not discarding the past. It's keeping the parts that really work for you and leaving the rest behind. When you're taking care of your health, you can still have the pleasure of enjoying your food. You can actually enjoy it more because it tastes delicious while you're eating it and fills you with energy and nutrition all the while.

Open Doors for Hope to Walk Through

One book that influenced me as a young man was *How to Eat to Live* by Elijah Muhammad, which spoke about the truth that our body is a temple. In religious culture and practice, the body is a sacred place, like it says in Corinthians 6:19, "Your bodies are temples of the Holy Spirit, who is in you."

Food is the source of how I feel every day. Feeling that love for myself is the fuel for making music. It's a practice of self-love and working on the self, part of who I am, building me towards operating in that higher self that I know we all are. It's the foundation of doing work for the people, doing work in the prisons for people that are incarcerated, building our community.

For my fortieth birthday party, my friends threw me a surprise party. These were people I am close with, and a lot of them are from Chicago. Lauren was there, too. We were talking about the violence in Chicago, and Lauren voiced her feeling that if we gave the kids better food, it would help stop the violence in Chicago because these foods and the things that we're giving them are creating an energy within them that drags them into a negative and violent space. When she said that, not everybody understood it. I thought it was brilliant. That's a pretty revolutionary way of thinking.

People think you stop the violence in just one way. What they don't know is that how we eat can be a component to bettering our communities and our families as well as ourselves. Food is a source for how we feel. Instead of coming down on people as a reaction to violence, we can start at the source. If you love yourself, if you truly have that feeling of pure love, you will never go out and destroy someone else.

My mother and I talk about this, about how you can't have a love for self and a love for human life and go out and take lives. My mom does some speaking, and she'll talk with communities where there is violence. One way she approaches these talks is to talk about love. The more we better ourselves and become clearer and healthier, the more we treat our bodies as temples, the better we become as human beings, and the better we are towards one another.

I used to have a temper that was different than it is today. I would pop off in an instant. But being conscious of my food helped me become more conscious of the responses my body had to people and situations. Eating foods that made me feel bad led to me being stressed out. Rather than being patient, I found myself lashing out from time to time. When what I was taking into my body changed, I could hear what my spirit and my intuition were saying because I had the energy to listen.

I started making these changes to my food when I was nineteen. More than thirty years later, I feel centered. I feel significant. I understand that time is short on this Earth, and I want to live the rest of my days as the best of my days.

"It's a positive force which guides my course," Brand Nubian says in "Dance to My Ministry." Later, he comes in with, "It's time to shine light, that's why I'm Provin' and Showin' / That the age has come to be conscious."

As someone who grew up eating burgers, pork, bacon—you name it, I ate it—I still find it incredible what changes in us and then changes us, and that all these many years later, I'm a person who is a vegan.

Am I saying that you should be a vegan? No. What I'm saying is that you have to do what's right for you, and only you know what that is. What people pursue doesn't need to be exactly what I pursued. For me, it was being vegan. For you, it might be something else. All I can do is tell you what I've done, to share the information I've learned from my teachers, to be open about the connections and changes I've made in my life. It's up to you to let the hope lead you. The only one who can make the choice for you is you.

When you choose to eat healthy, you're making space for good things to come to you. You're opening a door to a new way of feeling and being. You're creating an openness in the heart and in the body that you can fill up with joy, with creativity, with healthier relationships. You're removing the dust and the dirt, the things that clutter the mind and keep you from thinking clearly. Eating right for your body, feeding your body what you need at this point in your journey, can give you a clarity and a sharpness of mind to really be in tune with yourself and with your people.

That's a spiritual manifestation of a physical action, and one that can reset the way you experience your life.

PART 2

THE

BODY

" We all fly. Once you leave the ground, you fly. "

—Michael Jordan

Taking Flight

When I was twelve, I had a gig as a ball boy for the Chicago Bulls. My first role was at the bench, where I'd give the players water, and as they checked into the game, I'd get their warm-up suits and fold them. Eventually, I was promoted. My new job was making sure that the court was dry and safe for the players. I'd be there, courtside, ready and listening for the whistle to blow. When I heard it go off, I'd run out with my towel to wipe the sweat off the court. It was up close and real, life and breath and sweat.

I got the job because of a key introduction to the general manager of the Bulls while I was at an All-Star Game in Denver with my father, who played with the American Basketball Association. I didn't spend a lot of time with my father when I was young, and that has affected me throughout my life, but on this one occasion, we were out together, and he introduced me to the GM. When a job was mentioned, the GM said, "Write me a letter," and so I wrote and told him how dedicated I would be, and I got the job.

In 1984, I was there watching from the sidelines while Michael Jordan played his first season with the Bulls. I had never seen anyone do that with their body. It was like he was flying. I had been courtside with the Bulls before Jordan arrived, and when they drafted him, I could feel the change. The energy shifted. It was incredible, everything about it, from who he was and what he brought to how that translated to other people—the general manager and the coaches and everybody in the stadium. I could feel instinctively that it was the beginning of something, but I couldn't have told you of what back then. I couldn't see the future, but I felt the possibility all around me when I saw him play.

Like Jordan has said, "We all fly. Once you leave the ground, you fly."

I was thinking about all of this recently because a friend sent me a photo from that era that took me way back. It's a moment in a game, with two players in the air, head to head at the basket. Michael Jordan, who is in the early days of his career, is dunking on T. R. Dunn, who was already well-known for his stiff defense.

The note with the photo said, "Two Chicago legends in here." I wondered what he was talking about because Dunn was from Alabama and a player for the Denver Nuggets. As I scanned the image, I saw a young boy sitting there by the court, looking up at those men with the light on his face and an expression of awe. What my friend said, the way he presented that picture to me, touched something in me, because the kid in that image is me.

Looking at it now, I can see the little kid in that photo. He's dreaming of being something, just looking up at this person who is flying in the air, achieving their dream. Jordan was at the beginning of what he was about to become, and I'm seeing his greatness even in that space, a magnetism and a light and a power that he brought even before the world started to recognize it all the way.

The stands were not full yet. The whole audience hadn't caught on yet. Michael had, and I was there observing. That was the dawn for Michael Jordan. Those were the seeds for me. I see myself thinking how amazing he is, and that maybe, just maybe, I can also do something and be something.

That photo speaks to me so much, and it's beautiful. It was an energetic thing for me to revisit for myself because it actually made me realize that it was those moments and seeing people who were achieving at that level that allowed me to know that I could do it. I'm really dreaming and imagining what I can be, although I didn't even have the direction yet of what it would be. Not knowing what it is, but still looking to the future, with dreams and hope and motivation and inspiration.

When I look at the photo, I see myself witnessing Jordan's greatness. I see myself observing it by being around it, just sitting under that basket, watching this human being, a child of God, soaring in his power, soaring in his strength, soaring in his purpose. How physical it was, how spiritual it was. Just seeing him play ball, seeing all of them play, made me want to play ball at that level. I got my Air Jordan gear and a hoop on my closet door, and I'd jump in the air trying to jump like Jordan. I started working out so that I'd be better at the game, wearing weights on my legs so that I could learn to jump even higher.

I wanted to be able to move in that way.

I wanted to soar.

Let Your Light Shine

My life in basketball began when I was eight years old, playing in the Biddy Basketball league, where my uncle was a coach. The way the coaches managed the players was to send the best of us out in the first and fourth quarters. Those who weren't as skilled played in the second and third quarters. I was a second and third quarter guy, at first.

In one early game, they sent me out to play, and I scored no points, got no assists.

Back at the bench, I was crying because I had been kind of scared out there.

What I said was, "My stomach is hurting."

"Okay," said my uncle, and he let me be.

The next time we played, the same thing happened. They sent me out, I was scared and I scored no points, got no assists.

My uncle said, "What happened out there?"

My story about my stomach didn't play well this time. My uncle was not having it. He threw down his keys and started laying into me, and the gist of his rant was that I couldn't just give into being scared or feeling bad because if I wanted to be good at basketball, I was going to have to work at it.

In his way, he was giving me motivation. What he was saying somehow got through to me, and every day, before school, after school, I worked on my dribbling, worked on my game. Every day. It got to the point where my mother and my stepfather were tired of the sound of me hitting that ball, but I wanted it. I wanted to be better. I may have felt unsure on the court, but I could practice my dribbling and increase my confidence in this one area. As I kept at it, once I started getting into the games and doing some things, I had the feeling that doing this work was paying off. It came down to practice. That's it.

Once I had some of those skills, I could feel like what it was like to be on a team and watch the team grow. That was where my love for basketball really came in. I learned that I loved to play point guard. I liked passing the ball to set other people up for their shots. I felt like I could control the game and make sure everyone got a chance to touch that ball. I could tell when someone was hot, and pass the ball to them, and make that decision. Within playing basketball, I found my love for collaboration. Making sure everybody gets a piece. That even if you don't get that shot, when you're down the court the next time, I got you.

It was a community. There were lots of different guys on the team, people from different neighborhoods than mine. Some were more hood than I was; some of their parents had more money than mine. But we were always on the same team, and we had that bond of going out there and playing together to win. We saw the value of the support that we could give one another because when we all collaborated, we got better.

Basketball always brought that to me, and then it also brought the fun and the challenge of working on myself. In a sport, there's always somebody defending against you, blocking you from showing what you've worked on, trying to keep you from demonstrating your skill. It made me have to work harder, try harder. They might have been blocking me, but I learned that it's still about overcoming my own blocks. Whether it's dribbling, ball-handling drills, footwork, or conditioning for strength and speed, you've got to practice in order to get past the defenses. That's part of my love for the sport.

What I learned back then was that when I gave my body what it needed to succeed, I could get there. We all have things within us we want. You got to listen for that voice within you, telling you that you can get healthier, get stronger, try something new, try something different, express a part of yourself you haven't acknowledged out loud. When we're not doing as well as we want, it's not the other players keeping us from it, most times. It's ourselves, our own blocks, hesitations, fears, and shame. If you want to change, you have to find that motivation and get out of your own way, so you can see how bright you shine when you stop covering up your light.

Ask Questions

The same year I was a ball boy for the Bulls, I was known in my neighborhood for having a really big Adam's apple. It stuck way out of my neck, obvious to anyone looking at me, but to me, it wasn't anything I thought very much about. It was just a piece of me, a part of my body.

My godmother didn't feel that way about it. She took a long look at my neck one day and she didn't like what she saw. Instead of taking it for granted as natural, she saw it as something that was possibly wrong, and she turned to my mother and asked a question.

"Why is his Adam's apple so big?"

Followed by a firm suggestion: "You need to check his throat out."

Thank God she asked because when we went to the doctor, he said that I had a cyst that needed to be removed. I came out of the surgery with a series of stitches in my neck and a sense of relief because it was all going to be over now, and I could forget all about it. The doctor did warn me about being active while my stitches were healing up; I was to be careful and take it easy. On the list of forbidden activities was my favorite activity: playing basketball. But because I was a little boy who wanted to play ball, I did not follow that doctor's advice. I was not careful, and I did run around.

The result of all that running around was that the stitches from my surgery turned into a big keloid scar on my neck.

Choices change our bodies. This may have been the first time in my life that I saw this so clearly. Every time I looked in the mirror, that scar looked back at me, reminding me that if I had just listened to the doctor, I wouldn't have that scar. Everyone else could see it also, and my friends started to call me Cutthroat. I didn't like that at first, but eventually I embraced it. When I started embracing it, even when I heard them say it, "Cutthroat," it became a part of who I was. They still call me that, to this day. "Yo, Throat!" That scar, it's still with me.

So is what I learned from that experience.

As people, we are spirits that exist in these physical bodies, and there's so much about these bodies that contain us that we have no choice about. What you came into the world with, what was around you as an infant, none of that was up to you. Today, there's so much you can choose for yourself that will set you up for physical heath. Eating well, working out, avoiding cigarettes, getting that good sleep, drinking water, seeking relationships with health practitioners who can inform and support you. Making your well-being your priority is a choice.

Now I wonder what might have made a difference for me back then. What if the doctor had been a person I knew well, that I trusted? My physician now, Dr. Tracey, is a person whose advice I seek out because I respect her knowledge and perspective. She is a physician who studied both Western medicine and holistic medicine—what they call integrated medicine—because there is a place for all of it in her practice. She did her training with Andrew Weil, who, she said, always wanted it to be evidence-based.

She has so much to offer me, and her entrance into my life created a new foundation of care for me because having a relationship with a physician that I trust inspires me to be proactive about my health. I pay attention to my energy levels, to what I'm trying to accomplish in my life. I feel empowered to ask as many questions as I need in order to understand what I'm being promised in a medical setting.

Dr. Tracey believes that in order to be proactive about health, we have to take personal inventory. "You've got to sit down and think about what you want out of this process," she says. "You have to proactively think about what you're looking for because medicine is very personal. It's about being a part of the conversation."

She's taught me that the more I understand about who I am and what I need, the more I can ask for what I need, whether I want to build muscle to get ready for a role or keep my endurance up so that I can handle the pressures of life or have a smooth and steady voice so that I can say my lines up onstage and have the people in the audience not just hear me, but feel me.

She believes that patients need to ask questions and wants us to think about what it is that we really want before we go to see a doctor. She is always advising me to come in with that list of questions because you can't just rely on the doctor to be thinking about all the things that come up for you, or what you need personally to create a life of health for you. Distance runners need different medicine than construction workers; people who are raising children and always holding a baby on that hip are going to need different medicine than people who sit at a desk all day.

You've got to come in with awareness of what you do with your time, and what you want to do with your time. Dr. Tracey worked in a hospital setting for many years, and she will tell you straight out that most medical environments don't foster communication with patients. Hospitals aren't getting to know you when you check in. They're looking for a problem, fixing the problem, and telling you what to do. It's not a conversation. It's an instruction. If you want to have that conversation, one in which you are a *part* of the conversation, you have to come in with your questions.

Dr. Tracey sees a major disconnect when it comes to supportive communication between patients and providers. But you need that time, you need those answers: that's why you have to ask your questions.

This idea, that I have to ask, that I have the right to ask, has shifted the way I relate to going to the doctor, or the time I had to have tests run at the hospital. She empowered me to understand that there aren't any foolish questions, no matter what they are, and that if I want to ask, I should. People may feel very uncomfortable, but you can't even know what will be a really important detail unless you're open about your experience and what you need. Just put it out there because you don't know what seemingly small detail can be important.

A list helps. Write it down in advance, and bring it with you when you go to the doctor so that you stay focused. If you don't want to read it to them, you can just hand it over. Appointments are often scheduled one on top of the other, so if they are too pressed to answer, ask when you can make an appointment to discuss your questions. You can also ask about communicating with them digitally. If you can email them, it may be the nurse practitioner or a physician's assistant on the other end, but if they're in contact with the doctor, that can give you a little bit more time. The goal of insurance companies is to get patients in and get them out quick. If you want that extra time, you've got to be ready to ask for it.

Whoever you are, tell your provider what your habits and conditions are. For example, if you're looking at your computer screen all day, you need to tell your provider that because some of the advice out there isn't always practical, depending on your lifestyle and responsibilities. Health advice can include cutting down on screen time, but if your job means you're at the computer, you can't just cut down on that time. Health advice often asks us to sit less, but if your job requires you to sit all day because you're driving a bus, you can't decide to stop sitting. What do you do then? According to Dr. Tracey, there are always supportive options, but you can't find out unless you talk about who you are, what you need, and what is going on in your life. If you can't get off that computer screen, for instance, you can take your B vitamins and eat your healthy fats and oils because that lubricates your eyes. You can wear computer glasses. If your job is putting your eye health at risk, that's a conversation you need to have with your doctor. If driving too many hours a day is hurting your back, there are exercises you can do to support your back health. It's all part of taking inventory and then asking for that personalized support. That's what preventative health care is for.

It starts with asking the question. If you're not getting the results you want, Dr. Tracey says, "Whatever it is, if they're just saying you have to live with it, you should never accept that. Never. There's always something more that can be done. You keep asking until you get the answers that you want. You can't always change your position, but you can change the way you're looking at it. Sometimes life is about perception. Sometimes that can make all the difference."

As she explains it, Western medicine is so focused on triage. "I started out in emergency medicine," she said to me, "and now all of medicine is emergency medicine."

Dr. Tracey and I have spoken extensively about the limits of the Western medical system because it's about sick care. You go to the doctor when you're sick, get that medicine, and hope that's it. Western medicine asks, "What's wrong?" and "What type of disease does this person have?" Whereas lifestyle medicine asks the question, "What type of person has this disease? What can we do right? What does the whole person need?"

"There're some things that Western medicine can be very good at," she explains. "If you have pneumonia, you need to be treated. There are illnesses we can cure with antibiotics. If you're worried about what antibiotics can do, we can do things to mitigate that, like probiotics.

"There's a place for holistic medicine and a place for Western medicine. They can work together. You have to be informed. I want people to make informed decisions."

Traditional Western medicine is set up to diagnose problems. Lifestyle medicine takes a step back. It encourages you to think about your health not just when you get sick, but earlier, when you're still healthy. When you give yourself support along key areas, it will trickle down into your physical body to support your health for now and for years.

If you want to talk about being healthy, according to Dr. Tracey, that's where lifestyle medicine comes in. "When you've taken inventory, and you understand that your goal is longevity, or brain health, or you have a function in your life, like being an athlete, and you want to feel or be a certain way in order to do that. If you are dealing with something chronic, if you want to prevent and stop progression, holistic practices and alternative practices are looking at your whole self. If you want to talk about how you live, the choices you make every day, how to feel your best for the long-term, you need to find a practitioner who specializes in that, who has time to talk with you, to get to know you, not because something is wrong this very moment, but because you want to make sure you stay healthy."

When you're out asking your questions, you've got to be asking the right person. Not every doctor has the same training and awareness.

"You're not going to ask your plumber to fix the electricity," said Dr. Tracey. "You have to be in the right place at the right time."

When you call your internist because you're doubled over in pain, that's crisis mode. That's what Western medicine is very good for: diagnosing acute problems. If your appendix needs to come out, you go to the hospital. If you want to deal with an acute illness, you go see a specialist. The cardiologist is dealing with acute illness or chronic illness of the heart. They're there for triage, not for prevention.

Doctors do a lot of screening, but they're looking for certain thresholds. If they see that you may have diabetes, you'll be treated for diabetes. But what they're looking for are problems that can be fixed, a threshold after which you may need a medication. If you're healthy, you don't go to a cardiologist because there's really nothing wrong with you yet. When you're being proactive about your health, that's a different conversation with a different kind of practitioner.

When you're still healthy, that's the moment to initiate lifestyle changes—your food, your exercise, your stress—so that you don't become sick in the first place. That's where lifestyle medicine is useful because it focuses on nutrition, regular exercise, healthy habits, stress management, community, and sociability. It looks at the composition of the whole person. Ayurvedic medicine, Chinese medicine, other integrative practices, she believes, work better for long-term prevention and whole-person care.

Dr. Tracey isn't there to just react when I have a symptom. She's working with me to build up my immune system so my body will be at its peak, ready to respond for me. To do that, she works with me to understand who I am and what I need from my body so I can live at my fullest, which starts with me making an active effort to engage with my health and with health-related things. She's always encouraging me to tell her how I'm doing, where I'm at, what I'm thinking about.

One thing we talk about is longevity—how I can keep getting older in good form—because I don't want to take for granted that a sharp decline is inevitable. I know that as I get older, I want to maintain my strength, my ease, and my flow, mentally as well as physically. Everyone's always saying that as you get older, you're going to feel worse, you're going to look worse. That wasn't my experience, and I credit my lifestyle choices—from the workouts to the food that I eat. Yes, the body ages.

The poet Nikki Giovanni has some inspiring words about aging.

She talks about being sixty-five years old, feeling good, and enjoying her life at that age. She comes at it with a mindset of appreciation, and that's what I want to embody. As she says, "A lot of people resist transition, and therefore never allow themselves to enjoy who they are. Embrace the change, no matter what it is . . . It's completely liberating."

You have to be in the body you're in. You have to be present with who you are because even though you are so much more than a physical being, your body sets the stage for how you feel. Your body is how you move through this world and how you feel the world. Hands can play the piano or move a basketball up the court, arms can carry a child, legs can ride a bicycle to explore a new city.

Every day, I ask my body to do so many things for me. I ask it to deal with jet lag so I can be where I need to be, to wake up early in the morning so I can work out, to get to an early morning call time with energy to film all day, to perform with a complex range of emotion so I can deliver a character fully to an audience, night after night.

This body has carried me for more than fifty years, and I thank it, even while I ask it to keep carrying me forward, with health, with ease, with strength.

Self (Conscious) Love

The source of my lifelong physical esteem is not that time that I was named in one of *People*'s Sexiest Man Alive issues. It's the way the neighborhood guys made fun of me when I was a kid, and what I learned from those experiences about accepting all the parts of myself, even the ones that aren't beautiful to other people.

"Yo, Throat!"

Growing up on the South Side of Chicago, I saw that there was a lot of street life. People were on their porches, at the parks, on the streets, just going to the pharmacy, the liquor store, the record store. We all knew one another, we knew each other's families, we were raised around one another. It's community.

That meant that whatever your flaws were, people would talk about them, out loud.

I was made fun of for a few things. My height. My toes. My fingers. The scar on my neck. People would say things like, "Your feet are crazy. Your thumbs look so funny. You're so short." It was just out there. The other guys were always joking on me for being short, especially when they started getting taller, because until I was a sophomore in high school, I was five foot two. For comparison, my dad was six foot nine. Whatever your body looked like, whatever your physical flaws were, everybody around put them right out there. They would joke with me about my so-called flaws, but they let me know they still loved me, which meant that as a young person, I wound up feeling okay about my body, even the parts I was self-conscious about.

There was just no hiding, and shame comes from hiding. But say it out loud, and the feeling changes. You might be self-conscious, but you're owning it, embracing it. All that putting it out there helped me feel okay about whatever I didn't like. Even in the quirkiness of it and the differences of it, I still was able to say, "Well, that's what it is." It helped to have it put out there as a kid. I was forced into it, and it still helped me. You couldn't hide, you couldn't feel ashamed, it was just right out in the open, and the only thing to do was to accept it. The fact that we would discuss our flaws wound up being beneficial for me in terms of my body because early on, I learned to love those things about myself. No matter what, I still had love, so I was able to love myself.

I'm so grateful that throughout my life I have learned how to have love for my body, for what it looked like, for what it could learn to do, because we are continually having to get used to our new changes and physical quirks as we get older. In my twenties, I started going bald, and I felt very self-conscious about it. If I had still lived in the old neighborhood, I wouldn't have had much of a chance to avoid it—my friends would have been all over me, no room to hide. But as an adult, nobody was calling me out, and I did try to hide it, because my hairline receding made me feel older, and I didn't like that. I felt shame around it, so I would just put a hat on. I wore hats for years, until eventually, I realized I had to accept it because this was how God created me. I had to let it be and just make the best of it. That was the point where I felt good about it, and I was able to say, "Thank you, God. Thank you." That approach worked for me. Being bald turned out well for me, but I had to embrace it first.

That's the acknowledgment. Whether you feel bald, or short, or overweight, whatever it is, put it out there. You don't have to hide yourself, and you don't have to hide your insecurities. Everyone is insecure about something. In the end, some things about the body can be changed. Some are just with you. Whatever it is, you don't need to feel guilty or bad or negative about it. Just know where you are. Know who you are.

If what you are self-conscious about is the way your body looks or feels, you can make the decision to strengthen what can be strengthened, to tone what can be toned. Some things, like muscles, you have some control over. You can work out and grow your muscles if you want to, eat more protein, lift those weights. Anything else, you can change how you feel about it and how you see it. How tall you are is not in your control. Your hairline is not in your control. None of us stay twenty forever. Hair goes gray. We lose our hair. Everything changes. When you accept it and embrace it and love yourself because that is a part of self-love, you free yourself.

The body is more than how other people view you. It's what carries you through this world, the container of your spirit. It affects how you feel, and it is affected by how you feel, energized or tired, uplifted or depressed. It's how you experience the world. Ask anyone who is ill. It's not how you look that matters. It's what you can do with your body that counts.

That said, accepting our bodies as they are isn't easy. It's a process. I know because it's a process I went through. Now people will say, you're lucky you got a cool shaped head. And I think, you know, if I didn't, I'd find a way to deal with the shape of my head. I'd learn how to love all of me. It's not about the shape of my head or the size of my thumbs. It's that love for self that I got to find.

We all have something about us that's different, that we wish we could change. There's something about accepting it, embracing it, whether it's a scar or some stretch marks or you're balding. Once you embrace yourself, there's a beauty in everything. It's the hiding that's painful.

Like all those years when I wore those hats. When I look back at photos from that time, I'm always wearing a hat. You won't see any pictures of me during that time period without my hat. Now the hat's off. This is who I am.

Finding My Power

The first film role I ever stepped into was in a movie called *Smokin' Aces*, written and directed by Joe Carnahan and costarring Alicia Keys. My character, Sir Ivy, was a bodyguard, a no-nonsense individual who had a commanding presence when he walked on the scene, and according to Joe, I needed to be bigger to look the part. This wasn't anything I'd heard about before I signed on.

I was really excited for this role, but instead of feeling that rush of confidence, I had some self-doubt kicking around.

Not only did I need to look bigger to be believable as a bodyguard, I was going to have to use my strength because in one of the scenes, I learned, the script had me carrying Alicia down the stairs, and not just one flight. This scene was supposed to be intimate and strong and emotionally dangerous, not fraught with my insecurities about not being up to the task. And ideally, not physically dangerous for either of us.

You've got to remember that filming is all about repetition. It's not like one shot, you're in, you're out. Creating a scene that works for the director, that has the flow and the feel they're looking for is a numbers game. It doesn't happen just once. It happens as many times as it needs to get it right. That's hard enough when you're just speaking in conversation with another actor. When the scene at hand calls for walking downstairs, one staircase after another, and slowly, with another human being fully held in your arms—well, those arms can get really tired. I don't mind filming all day if it's the emotion that's missing from a scene, but there wasn't room for any mistakes here.

There was no way I was going to be the guy who drops Alicia Keys.

I was thirty-two years old. The last time I'd played organized sports, which was the last time I worked my body out in a programmatic way, had been fifteen years prior. I had been working on myself throughout all this time, but my focus was on my healthy eating and my spiritual growth. There were people around me who were working out, but I didn't choose to join them even when they invited me to workout with them. I wasn't trying to be buff because what I cared about was the spiritual. I learned how my eating related to how I felt in my spirit, but I still didn't understand that working out could have that same relationship with mind and soul. Because of that, I hadn't been engaging with the physical activities that contribute to bettering the body. I was still playing basketball, but there was no training, no lifting.

My secret weapon for preparation for this role was Harley Pasternak, a trainer who is a genius when it comes to nutrition and training. I put myself in his hands, ready to learn and get down with my fitness. I was grateful to be working with Harley because he's at the top of his game, and he's always coming through with that positive support. He really just had a way of communicating how beneficial working out would be and how it would only get better with time. He let me know that I would make it through, told me straight out that he knew that I could do this. Looking back, I understand how much taking in that mindset helped me persevere and succeed. Starting something new is exciting, but it's also terrifying. There's the adrenaline that comes from being challenged, and also that piece of you telling you that you can't do it. In order to get to that space where you feel comfortable and natural, you have to keep going.

When you begin a training program, or any kind of fitness

activity, you have to go in knowing that improvement is possible. You have to believe that wherever you're starting from, you can become stronger. You have to have faith that you can increase your endurance. Growth won't happen overnight, but if you keep going, it will happen. Those first few workouts can be intense, and you may need to take some breaks, but if you keep pushing through, the body will evolve. If you give yourself that chance to evolve, you will feel those changes, you will start to see those changes, and you will be amazed at what your body can do. Give it the time. Give it the effort. Do that for a while and you're setting yourself up to keep on going back, because experiencing the results is the best motivator there is. That's what I experienced, and every person you know who exercises regularly, that's the experience they're having, too.

You've got to start simple and then build up. We started with basic moves. I'd do eight to ten push-ups for four rounds and then repeat that progression with sit-ups, body squats, and lunges. We didn't work out for long hours each day. We just simply showed up for thirty minutes a few days a week. By being consistent and putting in the practice, I became stronger and better both physically and mentally. Over time, I got better, and I needed more, and my body wanted more. I learned that my body was good and enough, and that it wanted to grow. And that day of filming on the stairs—flight after flight after flight—I did not drop Alicia. (I don't know who was happier about that, her or me.) More than that, I felt really good about the progress I had made. Eventually I realized that the role in *Smokin' Aces* had been a real opportunity for me in so many ways, both as an actor and as an occasion to do all these things that were essentially me working on myself.

We all have reasons for making the change. Anyone you know who has started working out, there's something that sparks them to get up and get started. It could be an event that's coming up or something your doctor says to you. For me, it was a movie role, but truly, the movie was an excuse. I really wanted that for myself, too. I became so lit up by how good I felt when I worked out that I never wanted that feeling to go away. If you want to be lit up, you have to find your inspiration and then you have to make it yours and put your own energy into it.

I still hold the mentality that Harley gave me as a young man. I was in my thirties then, and he wasn't just focused on the moment, but on the lasting results. He used to say, "You're going to look better in your forties than you do now."

All these years later, I truly believe it. What he said came into fruition, even as the years pass. It is revolutionary to think that way because so much of what we are taught is the opposite. I was lucky to have that director send me to the gym to get me started because after *Smokin' Aces*, I trained with Harley for *American Gangster*, *Wanted*, and *Just Wright*. Even when I wasn't getting ready for a movie, I developed the habit of working out just for me because it had become my time to take care of myself in that way.

I've had a few trainers who have impacted my sense of how to care for the body. Harley was the one that put me on the track to understand what working out could give me for the rest of my life. I wanted to keep that light on, so I kept on training and going to the gym.

According to Dr. Tracey, we are made for movement and that movement oxygenates our cells. When you breathe into your lungs, the process by which the oxygen enters your bloodstream is called diffusion. Exercise increases diffusion, allowing more oxygen to reach the blood, which carries the oxygen to your cells.

We have arms and legs and we need to use them, Dr. Tracy told me. "The design determines the function," she said. "That means we need to move."

She acknowledges that lots of people have the kinds of jobs where they have to sit all day. If that's the case, you have to get up every hour because you have to be moving, she's said. The same goes if you're on a plane. Get up, move around.

"Exercise is medicine," Dr. Tracey said. "If exercise was a prescription drug, it would be the best prescription drug out there. There's no prescription drug on the market that can do what exercise can do."

She has listed them for me. Endorphins, serotonin, all the feel-good stuff that lowers your blood pressure, stimulates the relaxation response, lowers your stress—all that is in there. There's not one pill that can give you all that.

I've been working out for nearly twenty years now because I want to be fit, feel healthy, feel good about myself. I don't work out to be big or cut. I do it to have more energy. I want to be comfortable moving around and to feel flexible. I don't lift a lot of heavy weights, and when I do lift, I lift lighter and do more reps, which is more about getting the exercise in, taking care of myself, and getting that sweat. The connection I made over the years is that for me, the workout isn't about how my body will look when I'm done. It's about how it makes me feel. That's what keeps me going.

Progress, Not Perfection

In my early forties, when I was living in LA, I moved from Hancock Park to Beverly Hills, and I was looking for a gym where I could train. I wanted to find a place that was at the level where I felt that I needed to be, and I decided to try an Equinox that was right smack-dab on Sunset even though normally I would not like to be in the mix in that way. At the beginning, I stayed to myself, but as I would consistently go, this Equinox started to become a community to me.

That was where I met the people who trained me next. The first was a guy named Q, who approached me with the idea of working together. I'm not usually open to pitches from people I don't know, but with Q, there was a rapport. He loved hip hop and we connected around that. When Q moved away and I needed a new trainer, I had already developed a relationship with the head trainer at the gym, Yancy Berry. We had been connecting through the years in conversation, so I knew that I loved his energy. Music was one of the key places we connected because we're about the same age, and we would talk about hip hop and De La Soul and A Tribe Called Quest, all this music that we both loved. Since he grew up in the same era as I did, it was almost like we were from the same neighborhood, even though I'm from Chicago and he's from LA.

If you're going to have a trainer, you want it to be somebody who gets you, who gets what you're trying to accomplish and wants to help you get there. A good trainer can give you physical activities and exercises. A great trainer is going to take your goals and help you manifest them and motivate you throughout the process.

And Then We Rise
Workout Mix

◊

I work out five days a week. On my days off, I still feel great. It's the consistency of taking care of my body and sweating. Going in that gym, listening to A Tribe Called Quest and Big Daddy Kane and all the music that resonates with me. Just being in there, letting my mind go to wherever it needs to go. Not focused on whatever conversation I just had earlier. Not focused on the job I got to do today. Focused on me.

My mind goes to different places when I'm working out. The act of doing a side plank and then reaching to the sky, or doing mountain climbers, where my knees touch my elbow—when you're focused on making contact like that, there's no time to think about other things. It's hard to be working out and be drifting off. It's a moment where you just got to be present. There's just something about that time that gives me time.

When I play nineties hip hop, I get a charge. It's what I love to work out to. It's my music, the music I grew up with, and it takes me back while it centers me in the moment. Listening to the songs on this playlist, I feel their power, and I have that feeling that I can achieve and accomplish anything. It's the motivation I need. The words reaffirm who I am and how great I am and bring up conscious things that resonate with me and get me going. As hard as the beats are, and as raw as some of the lyrics are, it's a comfort. It's a motivating factor that embraces me and pushes me to bring my best.

"Microphone Fiend," Eric B. & Rakim

"Set It Off," Big Daddy Kane

"I'm Still #1," Boogie Down Productions

"Top Billin (Acapella)," Audio Two

"Take It Personal," Gang Starr

"How Many MC's . . . ," Black Moon

"Scenario (LP Mix)," A Tribe Called Quest

"Rock Dis Funky Joint," Poor Righteous Teachers

"You're a Customer," EPMD

"They Want EFX," Das EFX

"Livin' Proof," Group Home

"The Choice Is Yours (Revisited)," Black Sheep

"DWYCK," Gang Starr and Nice & Smooth

"All for One," Brand Nubian

"Straighten It Out," Pete Rock & CL Smooth

"Represent," Nas

"Unbelievable (2005 Remaster)," The Notorious B.I.G.

"Come Clean (E New Y Radio)," Jeru the Damaja

"Passin' Me By," The Pharcyde

"I Got It Made," Special Ed

"Stop, Look, Listen," MC Lyte

"Slow Down," Brand Nubian

"Sound Bwoy Bureill," Smif-N-Wessun

"Next Level (Nyte Time Mix)," Showbiz & A.G.

"Shut Em Down (Pete Rock Mixx)," Public Enemy and Pete Rock

"The World Is Yours (Tip Mix)," Nas, Q-Tip

"Brooklyn Zoo," Ol' Dirty Bastard

"Uptown Anthem," Naughty by Nature

"Just Hangin' Out (2017 Remastered)," Main Source

"One in a Million," Pete Rock & CL Smooth

"Tonight's da Night," Redman

"Rebel Without a Pause," Public Enemy

"Know the Ledge," Eric B. & Rakim

"Award Tour," A Tribe Called Quest

"Ego Trippin' (Part Two)," De La Soul and Shortie No Mass

"One to Grow On," The UMC's

"93 'til Infinity," Souls of Mischief

For as long as I've known Yancy, he's been a life coach. I was getting that from him through osmosis, because when you're training, you still talk about life. It's like the way your hairdresser or barber is like a therapist because you're having these conversations with them all of the time. Yancy and I talked about goal setting; he has a great approach to that. "Who do you want to be? How do you want to show up in the world?" he asked. "Take a look at all the different parts of your life—relationships, health, business, every aspect. What are things you want to do, to accomplish, to have? Think about it like you were a kid, with a sense of exploration and fun. Now ask yourself, what is the most important part of all of these? What do you want to work on?"

I'm impressed by Yancy because he's always in a positive space. I don't like being around or staying around people who always bring up the negative. Yancy is the antithesis to that. During the pandemic, we would work out on Zoom, and I would think, *How is he staying positive every day?* I was working on staying positive, but he was positive every day. He's going to find the light, no matter what. If I'm working with a trainer who is just all about trying to be Hollywood and trying to get these girls and just about his Instagram or her Instagram, that's not going to work because that's not the direction I'm going, and those are not my goals. That's not the energy that I want to take in every day.

Yancy—I call him Sir Yance, as in, Sir Yance-a-lot—he's just a really good, levelheaded human being who happens to be a high-level trainer. He's a guy who is willing to grow; he's humble and also a leader and someone who knows all about growth, perseverance, and dedication. People have always gravitated towards him because he has this way of bonding with you.

Yancy is often the first person I have an intimate conversation with in a day because I usually work out early in the morning. You have to ask yourself, *Who is that person?* The people that you are constantly in communication with, you're taking in their energy, and you're absorbing their thoughts.

I talked with Yancy about his belief in partnership, groups, and teamwork. "You're going to be so much more likely to succeed in anything that you want to do if you have a strong partner," he said.

Yancy is about so much more than the physical. He believes that to be a strong human being, you also have to focus on the emotional and spiritual aspect, whether you have a family goal, a creative goal, a community goal. "Some people think that wellness, emotional and spiritual well-being, therapy, that they're not tough," he said. "When the truth is, it's the most tough! It's the most powerful thing in the world to take care of yourself, your physical and spiritual and emotional well-being."

Even as someone whose professional career is built on helping people develop physical strength, he knows that what's internal is what matters first, and then after that, the external comes. "What you accomplish internally, as far as emotional health and well-being, happiness, joy, these things are more important than external things," he said. "They will also lead to the external things. That's been my experience. The more fulfilled and happier I get, the more confident I get internally, and these external goals, not only are they more accomplishable, but I actually enjoy the process a lot more."

That's a space where we completely agree.

One thing I've learned from Yancy is that the way to progress is not about seeking perfection. It's about the practice. Working out has become another way of feeding myself and giving myself love. My workout time is my time. It's for me. It is so valuable in the process of me becoming a better person, a greater person, just because I always make sure I lock that time down for me.

Yancy and I talk about how wellness extends from self, outwardly, affecting everything. "It's not just physical health," he says. "It's not just being able to work out and lift weights or be able to run, but it's emotional wellness, it's intellectual wellness, it's even social wellness and the health of our community."

Yancy and I have been working together for more than five years now, and a lot of our training has been functional training, which I love. That, to me, is some of the most important stuff—that and tightening my core. I was often getting injuries from playing sports, and since I've gotten my core to this place, I'm not getting injured, even as I've gotten older. That's why I work. If I don't have the time, I make the time. If there's a morning where I need to leave by six, I might get up at four to work out, or I'll work out in the afternoon.

That's why I always make sure that I go to the gym to get my body moving, even if I'm not in the mood. We all have those moments where it's more tempting to just stay in bed or take the day off. When you're getting into fighting a workout routine, some days it's not going to go well. You might feel like you might try to skip out on it, or you might not feel like doing it, or it just might not turn out the way you want it to. It might take longer than you thought to see any type of results. You've still got to do it because that's the only way those results will show up.

Even when I don't feel like it, I'll still do the workout, and thirty minutes later, I'm so glad I did. I don't always want that workout, but I always need it. When I have meetings all day, the workouts don't take my energy away, they give me the energy to get through it all, as myself.

I'm always happier after that workout, and I promise you this: You will never regret that choice to work out. You will never regret figuring out what your body needs to feel amazing. Getting back into the gym at thirty-two—after fifteen years without really working out—was a moment of change for me, a beautiful change that came with the discovery that when I work out, it gives me energy, and I can keep that energy burning. I started for a role. Now I do it for me, so I can take it out into the world and feel good moving through the rest of my life.

The way you feel after a workout, that's the space of psalm.

Finding the Light

The pandemic wasn't only one thing for me. There were so many layers to it. There was the concern and worry I had for my community because Black people were affected so strongly and disproportionately, both in terms of health and economics. There was an aspect of personal growth because for the first time in a very long time, I had the space to be still and learn more about who I was. And then I got Covid myself, and it took a very long time for me to feel well again. During this era, like many people, I thought a lot about health and about illness. Getting sick affected me physically and it impacted me mentally. I had brain fog that made it hard to recall certain things. My mind felt like it wasn't fully functioning in the manner to which I was accustomed. It was a scary feeling and a very frightening time in my life. Each day I would ask myself,

Do you feel better? Is your mind clear? I kept waiting and hoping that I would get that energy and clarity back.

I know I wasn't alone in being out of tune with my spirit. Everybody was dealing with Covid differently in our own realities, but what we all experienced together was a deep sadness.

One morning, I called my therapist to say that I was having a hard time getting out of my head, and that I felt depressed and anxious in a way that I hadn't experienced before. She was talking to me about changing my mindset and understanding that this is not where I'm going to be forever, encouraging me to give it time, to just stay in the God space. I was trying to hear her, but the fear was taking over.

I turned to the body to see if working my physical aspect could influence this feeling that I couldn't seem to shake. I put on A Tribe Called Quest and started doing some push-ups inside because it was raining outside, breathing really hard and feeling like my head was about to burst. I felt a pressure and a tension that I hadn't felt before, an overwhelming emotion.

It was a spiritual bout, a spiritual fight, a mental fight, all rooted in the physical, because I had been sick, and I still wasn't feeling completely better.

I thought, *Should I cancel this workout?* But I knew that I decided to work out in the first place because in those shadowed moments, sometimes the way through is mental or creative, through speech or song, and sometimes it is physical, through sweat.

"I can do it," I decided. "I'm going to go make it through."

I wasn't in the best space because I was feeling so vulnerable, but even though the fatigue was there alongside me, an unwelcome visitor, I pushed through it and I got it done.

There's a reason I've spent so much energy developing these tools. All the scriptures that I read, the mantras I say, the dedication I have to working out, my determination to be proactive about my health. It's all to find that light again when I'm feeling the darkness. It's all to lift myself back up.

It's even better when I can share the experience with other people.

One thing that lifted me up during this challenging time was connecting with the world online through working out, listening to concerts, having spiritual conversations, you name it. I created a show called *Com + Well*, a health and wellness series on YouTube that highlights conversations with my friends and teachers about self-care and wellness. One of the episodes features Yancy and me talking about fitness and doing a workout together. You can access it on YouTube if you want to train with us.

I got so much joy out of doing these online workouts with other people. Caring for the self has so much power when you're in a community of other people who are also working on themselves. It just creates a shared energy that reverberates around, feeding everyone who is involved.

That's why we also launched a live workout series on IG Live. I was hearing from people across the country who were saying that they started working out because they saw how many other people were doing it, too, and they joined us. "I did it," the messages said. "I did it at my own pace, at my level, and I did it."

By coming together with a spirit of feeling better, together, the energy flowed through and around and back again, lighting us all up, reminding us that we were all in it together.

Start Simple

I know what it's like to begin training again after years of inactivity. In my experience, the beginning should be simple so you can let the feeling of it all sink in. Get out for a walk. Have a few glasses of water. Easy as that. Dr. Tracey and I talked about physical health, and she said that people can have a tendency to overthink exercise. Walking is great, and so is fast walking and bicycling. You want to get moving, and the more you do, the better.

If your goal is improvement, aim for progress, not perfection. Small, incremental gains. If you work on getting better by making one improvement every one to two weeks, Yancy told me, you are very likely to be successful.

WEEK ONE

According to Sir Yance, you want to use the first week to build in the habits. Write down how you are becoming active, write down what you eat, write down what you drink. Write down all the things, all the time. From there, every week you can make an improvement little by little. No matter what it is you're eating, eat whatever you are eating, do whatever you're doing for exercise now, but be sure to write it down so that you can be aware of where you are at and what needs to change. Like he said, your first week's progress can be just writing it all down.

If you're ready to get moving, start with walks. Drink more water. When you see yourself sticking with that, momentum will help you want to keep going.

WEEK TWO

If you want to change your body, start with your food—75 percent of body change is diet. Figure out your nutritional aspect. Make an improvement in your diet. You can start by taking vitamins every day. This is something simple. A multivitamin gives you things that your current diet may not be providing or what your body can't produce to the degree that you need it.

One of the best things you ever want to do, if you want to improve your eating, is to send your journal to an accountability partner every single day. Your accountability partner could be any other human being who is a supportive human being. Write down every single thing you eat every day, send it off in an email or a note, every single day. It's all about progress and accountability.

How do you want to feel? What do you want to achieve? For your physical body, do you want to be more limber or do you want to be stronger? If you're walking, you can start adding distance and time to your walk. You can increase your pace. To limber up, incorporate some very basic bodyweight things like stretching. Try to stretch in a way that doesn't injure you. Start to stretch and move your body. To get stronger, do things like bodyweight squats. Do push-ups or sit-ups or forearm planks.

WEEK THREE

This week, continue to think about your goals and build on the movement aspect while you stay aware of what you are eating and drinking. A great move is to change your snacks. If you are somebody who tends to eat cookies or chips, switch to fruits or vegetables.

You can begin to include some more focused training or workouts. Hit the street and keep that walking going. Pick up the pace and get your sweat on. Get down to the local gym and learn from the people there. Check out some of the workouts online if a gym isn't accessible to you. There are so many workouts offered online that everyone can find something that speaks to their skill level, energy level, and what they want to get out of it. If you want to do some moves with me and Yancy, check out *Com + Well* on YouTube. We've also included a rundown of our workout on page 89.

WEEK FOUR

Keep journaling, keep up with your vitamins, keep honoring yourself through movements, and be conscious of what you're putting into your body.

If you've been walking consistently, you can incorporate light weights. Walk holding your five-pound dumbbells or with ankle weights. You can increase your speed into light jogging. Move into a more challenging form of exercise: use your body weight to squat, then start doing squats holding a dumbbell. Keep going to the gym. Keep doing those online workouts. Keep learning about what your body needs.

Remember:
The goal is not perfection, it's progress.

Yancy Berry's Beginner's Full-Body Workout

At the back of this book (page 208), you'll find a link to the *Com + Well* episode in which Yancy and I do our Spidermans and our squats. You can join us there, or if you're off the grid for the moment, here's the kind of workout Yancy will take me through at sunrise on any given morning.

WARM UP

20 to 25 seconds each exercise

- Neck circles
- Swim backward
- Swim forward
- Chest open and close
- Side-to-side twists
- Hip circles
- Bodyweight squats

WORKOUT

4 rounds of the below circuit

Upper Body

10 to 12 Spiderman push-ups

Modification: kneeling Spiderman push-ups

Core

30 to 60 seconds side plank

Modification: side plank with knees down

Lower Body

10 to 12 squat jumps

Modification: deep bodyweight squat

Start Where You're At

If you're a beginner and you walk into an advanced workout, odds are you're only going to be able to do a slice of it because it's just not made for you. That's okay. That's just how it is. I have a friend who does a lot of running, a guy who did half-marathons, who would run twelve miles a day. When I tried to join him on a run, I was way back there because I was just starting. I may have gotten to five miles. That's okay. I have to give myself credit for trying. Is the story that I could only do half of what he did? Or that I made it to five without having a history as a runner?

As much as I wanted to do what he could do, as much as I'm a person that wants to excel and wants to be at the highest level of achievement, I recognize that if I want to get there, I have to start where I am. Your highest level is not the same as somebody else's. Starting where you are, aiming for your highest level, that's what it's about. The questions to ask yourself are, *What is my highest level, and how do I continue to evolve?* Not, *Why can I not do what these other people are doing?*

Stopping where you are is part of starting where you are. It's not the same as giving up. If you know you can get to the finish line, push yourself. Stopping too soon is the same thing as cheating yourself. If you have the training and you don't want to do the work, that's a different thing. If you're just starting, be honest with yourself about the level you're at. Perform at your own level and create the challenge that is right for your level, nobody else's.

There was a day I'll never forget when my daughter, Omoye, and her friends and a friend of mine, Rahsaan, came through and we all worked out together. Rahsaan lived down the block from me when I was a child; I've known him since I was five years old. It was in high school that we really became close. He's one of my best friends, one of my greatest friends, the strongest of friends, one of those friends that keeps you grounded. I can talk to him about a lot of different things in life because he just knows me. We balance each other out.

Omoye and her friends had been out the day before having a nice time, so when they worked out they were tired and hungover, but they still decided to go for it because they wanted to do this for themselves. The day before, Rahsaan and I were drinking, too; he was kicking it, and he still came out and did it. We were doing climbers, oblique work, intense work.

Rahsaan did what he could do and then he went to lay down and rest. He must have done half the workout before he hit the couch.

When we finished, we took the mats in and put up the weights, and I said to him, "Hey, man, good job. You did good." I was happy for him because he got it in. He started where he was, and he did it.

When I said that, he shared with me that it moved him in a positive way because he was getting support and affirmation. What he thought I would say was, "Hey, you quit during a workout; you couldn't do it." I didn't see it that way at all. What I saw was him doing half of it instead of none of it.

I hope that my response gave him fuel and inspiration to feel like the next time, the next workout, he would go further. We all need motivation, like I got from my uncle, although a delivery of gentleness and compassion goes a long way, too.

"You didn't do all the reps? That's okay. You did the reps you did. You can do more tomorrow."

That's the attitude I want to have with my people. That's the attitude I want to have with myself.

How we talk to ourselves really is super important. Why say to yourself, *I should have done two miles?* How about, *I did one mile. Tomorrow I'm going to try to get in a mile and a half.*

People think that if you're given a workout, even if it's the first workout, you're just going to come in and perform at the instructor's level. That's just not realistic. You can try, you might be able to, but if you don't do it all, that's okay.

The instructor does this every day! That level is the goal. It's not the beginning. You've got to know where to meet yourself, wherever you are.

If you go to the point where you can say, *I'm giving my all to this, and I know I gave my all,* be happy. Give it your all. Give yourself a chance to see what you can do. Practice. As you keep going, and you continue, a week later, two weeks later, three weeks, a month, you're going to see the effects. You've got to be faithful that you are doing the work, and that work is going to create the change.

Welcoming Joy In

When I started working on myself, I was able to begin fulfilling my happiness and feel full of that happiness. What I've gotten from all of this self-care of my body is a feeling that I want to keep. I accept that, lifelong, I'm going to continue to create and be a part of happiness and joy. That's what I envision. That's what it's going to be. This is what I am created to be. This is who I am. This is what it is.

I had to work on the things that I was ignoring, the patterns that weren't helping me that I kept repeating in my life. I had to investigate all that pain that I pushed away that I didn't want to feel. The way I see it now is that you can trudge your way through or work your way through, but you still have to go through. We can keep on in a way where we walk with all the weight on our shoulders, or we can try dealing with the bad stuff and peeling it off. If you feel a nail in your foot, are you going to keep walking with it in there because you're tough? What if you actually pulled the nail out?

I've had a lot of happy moments in my life, but it's not perpetual joy. Even though I know I'm taking care of myself, that I'm focused, I will feel sad at a moment, whether something big has happened that I am grieving or my mind is taking me to a place of hardship. I'll always remember finding out that my cousin passed away in a car accident, and less than fifteen minutes later, I was up onstage performing. I performed even though I was sad, and after I got off the stage, I still had to go through those feelings. I still had to do the work to find that good space again. What keeps me going is that I know that when I push through it, I get to another place. What keeps me going is my hope for my own future.

My journey continues, and I know it isn't done. It isn't a place of arrival, it's a space of continual processing and learning. I still go through moments where I wonder what I'm doing and what it all means. I find myself thinking, *What is my life? When I transition, will my life have meant something?*

The more work we do to find that light, the more that light stays with us even in times of darkness. That's been my experience. How do you experience joy? When great things are happening in your life, do you imagine that they'll soon disperse or go away? Doing this work to grow, continually, I've started coming to understand that this work of giving myself love is my way of life now. The choice and the discipline is what led to the actual practice of it, and one day, it hit me: This is how it is. This is really how I'm going to feel continually. These beautiful things that I've been attracting in my life with this new way of being are going to keep coming.

The same is true for you. The future is a new place where anything is possible if you truly have love for yourself and if you're willing to keep trying again and again. As long as you're here on this planet, you can choose to take this journey.

When you take steps to love yourself in that way, even just for a few weeks, and you start to feel how good you feel, remember, it's still just the beginning. Six months in, you'll feel it even more. Yes, you'll still hit the tough spots because you're human. You'll also know that you can handle it because you've seen how it all compounds. You've started to recognize your power. And you'll just know: there's going to be more of this. It's going to keep coming for you, as long as you invite it in.

Your life is supposed to be an abundance and happiness and joy and health and friendship and laughter, even during the ill moments that happen in life, even during the painful moments. You are going to experience them, and you will have to deal with them, and you'll also have the overriding love to come through.

You were created for joy and power. It's what you are meant for and what you are worthy of. That's who you are, and that's what it is.

PART 3

THE
MIND

" Riding through the city with the top down. We ain't got no ceilings to our thoughts now. It's a beautiful ride. "

—August Greene, "Black Kennedy"

Keep Your Head to the Sky

"Well, let me tell you about a trip a time ago . . ."

So begins the first line of the first rap that I ever wrote. I was twelve years old, visiting my cousin Ajile in Ohio. Ajile knew some guys who had a crew called the Bond Hill Crew who were a few years ahead of us, like older brothers. They would perform at skating rinks and do their gigs, which was really impressive because they made it. For us, they were like the Run DMC of Cincinnati.

It was because of these guys that I felt that pull of inspiration to create my own lyrics. Instead of watching TV, I went upstairs to the bedroom to see if I could also write a rap. It was an electric moment because what flowed out of me felt like I was tapping into something alive and full of possibility, and when I rapped it to myself, I thought it sounded pretty good.

> *Well, let me tell you about a trip a time ago . . .*
> *I was going there to run a cold blooded show.*
> *When I was there, I saw some people jamming too.*
> *They called themselves the Bond Hill Crew*
> *Dr. Ice, Romeo and Master E.*
> *All of the Bond Hill Crew wrapped into A-T*
> *I asked him, could they rock with me?*

These lines tell the story of the moment and about my connection to these guys. I don't remember all of what I wrote, but I do recall clearly how it felt to write it and to share it. When I rapped my lyrics to them, they embraced it, loved it, and encouraged me. The way they kept saying, "Damn, this is good . . ." is a vivid memory. That exchange of energy, me giving that rap to them, and how they reacted to me, made me feel like, *I am something. I have something to give. I have something that I feel good about.*

The whole experience fired up something deep within me. It was my earliest introduction to the divine nature of creating, and it's a part of what set me on my path. Using my mental energy in this way—to produce, to imagine, to call forth these words and rhythms—was so uplifting for me. My brain was fully engaged. My heart was filled with intention.

When I'm freestyling today, that energy is there with me. It all comes from the love I have for rap music. It was true back then and it still is to this day. Creating is such a spirit, heart, pure, divine thing to do, and I rejoice in it. When you're creating, you hope and work and believe. You do it from a place of true love, an openhearted place that allows you to be free within your own imagination. Creativity is a space of self-examination and self-expression, a space to release negative thoughts along with positive hopes, to take energy that's bottled up inside you and allow it to emerge in a fruitful and beneficial way. I'm not always aware of exactly what I'm thinking when I'm writing my lyrics. It's emerging from my subconscious, coming through me. It's of me more than it's by me.

Experiencing those feelings within my creative process, I just know that it's God's work, connecting me to my purpose. I am grateful for what led me to it, and I have gratitude that I chose to go that way. Creating, using the mind and the imagination that God gave me, allows me to fully feel myself and know my power. It's what I meant in the lyrics of a song I wrote for August Greene—a project I was blessed to work on with two amazing creators, Robert Glasper and Karriem Riggins. I wrote, "Riding through the city with the top down. / We ain't got no ceilings to our thoughts now. / It's a beautiful ride."

When you create, when your mind connects with what is outside of you, when your brain is focused on translating what you've been absorbing so that you can release it in a different form, whether that form is based in sound, language, or images, it's a special thing. It's truly a beautiful ride. It's a mind trip. It's a soul trip.

When I wrote that first rap, the music came from me. They didn't tell me to write anything, but I was moved to do so because receiving their creativity lit me up. I felt something in my spirit and in my heart that I wanted to express because it was a true exchange of creative energy. When I used that moment to really write my own material, it was like electricity passing from one body to another. I felt their power, and I felt the power within myself of being able to say my raps. I was watching their reaction, wondering if they would like it. I was expressing myself to them, and when they gave me feedback, when they appreciated it, when they said, "Oh, this is dope," that gave something to me. It all started because they were out there sharing their own creative impulses and style, and as I took that in, it showed me what was possible for me.

People talk about visibility. Seeing people out in the world looking the way we look, doing how we do, creeps into how we think about what we can do. To see it, to be able to dream it, to envision it. How else do we imagine things but by seeing something that sparks the next thought? The imagination is not a camera. It doesn't need to see something specific in order to reproduce it. But the raw materials that we take in become food for our imaginations. Sometimes what we're absorbing through our experiences is founded in joy. Sometimes it's founded in pain. It all becomes food for our minds and our creativity.

Being an artist is a journey and a path. I started with that rap when I was twelve, then I was making music in my neighborhood, and at nineteen, I came out with my first album. When that happened, it wasn't like all my reviews were just so great and I was clearly on the way to becoming a well-known artist. It's not always like that. I wasn't getting national radio play and recognition. I just came out and released the music, and some people knew who I was, some people didn't. Some people didn't care. Some heard it and weren't into it. I kept wondering, *What can I do to get better?*

The first time I realized I could win awards, I was twenty-six years old, and some friends of mine, the Roots, were up for a Grammy, in competition with some of the most popular artists, from Puff Daddy to DMX. When the Roots won, I had this moment with it, that feeling of, *Man, I can do it.*

Years later, I did do it. It took a lot of work to get there. I'm still always wondering, *What can I do to get better?* I still want to perform at my highest level, in my art and in my actions, in my relationships to myself and my interactions with other people.

That's why all these things that we're talking about in this book are so valuable to me. My food puts me into a space where I feel calm and energized. Working out takes me to that place of being in the moment. Relaxation lets stress out of my body. A calmed mind can process what life is throwing at me. Art and music let me be inspired and feel that divine expression. Therapy gives me space to process my feelings and gain self-understanding. God gives light to my soul.

Together, all these aspects give me the foundation to manifest my dreams at the highest level.

Creativity Is Divine

When I'm creating, I'm going to the deepest parts of myself, trying to discover ways to connect with other human beings. It's a challenge for me to describe my process of creativity verbally because it's something that happens deep within me, in a place where words diffuse into something more like sensation. Creating is truly a connection with God, an allowing of a higher power to come through you and express itself creatively in whatever medium you are drawn to. When I get out of the way, when I stop judging it and putting my ego to it, when I allow it to just come through, that's when I am creating at my best.

I started my journey as an artist with my music; later on, I began acting in film and then television. I knew that I wanted to act in a Broadway play someday, but it took time to get there. Getting to a place is not always about that one big leap. More often, it's a series of baby steps.

My earliest exploration of theater as an adult was right before the pandemic, as a part of the Audible series called *Words + Music*, which features artists performing songs and speaking alongside the music. I wanted to create something that would feel fresh, that would combine theater and music. This piece would be my first time writing something that was a dialogue-driven performance, along with a sequence of songs.

Awoye Timpo and NSangou Njikam, two vibrant and thoughtful people with whom I already collaborated on live shows, agreed to participate, and together, we sat in my apartment and threw all of these various ideas and stories up on the wall. The possibilities were all around me.

The inspiration for the performance that we created came from a walk I took through a labyrinth at Miraval, a resort in Arizona, where I moved slowly and consciously around this winding circle in the desert, centering and calming myself. At the end of my walk, I encountered a bluebird. Seeing this bird, I had the strong feeling that my father was speaking to me through this bird, giving me a sense of peace and security and letting me know everything was going to be okay.

Bluebird Memories is about my growth as a human being and my journey of learning who I am. In this piece, I am speaking to my father, who transitioned into the afterlife in 2014. I talk about how I miss him, recalling things I learned from him, sharing the ups and downs, the story of how I became an artist, and how grateful I am. As I speak, the conversation leads into songs.

We recorded the performance, and we presented it live as a one-man play with a live band. Audible gave us a great theater in New York, Minetta Lane, intimate and beautiful. I was excited to invite friends and nervous at the same time; it was a really incredible experience for me. It was healing and it was powerful, and I consider it to be one of my best expressions as an artist.

Experiences like this are why I value and appreciate my creative aspect even more at this point in my life than I ever have before: because I understand that creativity puts divinity into practice. It is a place of growth and self-discovery. It allows us to deal with and heal from the harder parts of life. To live in emotion and beauty and be present in that. To become more powerful individuals and to be lovers of self. It's one of the most divine ways that human beings can connect and express and receive one another.

I know there are a lot of people out there trying to get to where they're going, working to come up in their way, and it doesn't always happen the way you want it to, the way you hope it will. If that's where you're at, remember that when you're operating in your purpose, when you're holding your vision, if your goal is to reach more people, you've got to keep at it and keep working at that vision and craft and figuring out the ways. Whatever you're struggling with, remember, it might be your first try. It isn't going to be your only. Yet we put so much pressure on everything—like it's the one thing that's going to make or break us.

You have to remember the joy. You have to feel confident in your work. To prepare. To remember that you can do it, that you're supposed to be here doing this. If you've been doing it for years, and you're going to keep doing it until you stop breathing on this Earth, then you know what your purpose is. The way you want to be recognized and seen will happen at the time that it's supposed to, but you've got to make sure you're doing your part. As long as you're seeking and working at your goal and vision and you know you are giving your best self, then God is seeing that and knowing, aligning everything for it to happen for you when it should.

You've got a whole path. Give your best. Know that when people celebrate it, that's great, but you're still going to be wanting to do more. Just stay on this path, and know you're giving your best. Keep at the craft of it, keep taking what is needed for your spirit, for you to deliver.

If art is your path, I do believe that whatever you do, if you're doing it with love, if it's something you do innately, naturally, passionately, then doing it is productive and fruitful for society and people. Just by doing it, you're putting that love out there. That's what I'm trying to do as an actor. As a musician, too. Those are two things I can say that I do in my career that I want to do.

Remember that God put you here for a purpose. However hard it's been, it'll all be worth it as you travel through this. You never know what this preparation is building you up for.

When you create from a pure place of love and imagination, if you're putting it out there, some people might not like it. It might not speak to them. They may have their own experiences. They might not rock with it or it just might not be their taste. Some people don't like chocolate. Some people don't like jazz. You've got to take that into consideration when you're being creative.

If you're a musician and you're creating your music and it isn't hitting the way you'd like it to, that's painful. If you're a script writer, and you want to sell your script, it's painful when it isn't received. If you're an artist creating paintings or sculptures, it's painful when people don't get it. I think it's important to recognize that you can come from a pure place and not get that immediate recognition from other people. There's still that space where, if you've come from that place of love, imagination, and expression, there is value in what you're doing. It can take time for other people to recognize it. It can take a hundred rewrites to get there. It can take a hundred songs, a hundred auditions, a hundred canvases.

Whatever you do, the process might be kicking you in your ass, knocking you over and all that, but you've been through enough experiences to be able to bring it. It's not easy. Who can put a time on when it's going to happen for you? I often have to remember to give myself some grace. That's what you've got to do if you're working to create and to share your artistry with other people. You can't beat yourself up. Instead, give yourself love and encouragement. Find those tools and resources that help you deal with the pressures. We don't know how long life will be, and as long as we're here, we can remember that our purpose is to create something beautiful, and to do it from a pure place of love.

I always acknowledge the divineness of creativity. If you believe in a higher power and the creation of the world, that the creator created the world, that's where creativity came from. From the power to create a universe and the Earth and heavens and the birds in the sky. When we create, we are connected to that divinity, and to all other human beings.

Not everything in life is about being appreciated by other people. When you're walking outside and you see a tree, it's a tree whether or not you stop to appreciate its beauty. Does it need your approval to be beautiful? Does it need to look just like the other trees? Does it need you to marvel at it in order to be its full expression of itself? It's a tree. It's beautiful in its own way, and it's rooted in its own space. It's what it's supposed to be.

Whatever anyone else says, creativity that comes from that pure place of love in your mind and imagination is divine.

Think on These Things

Dr. Tracey and I talk about gratitude and forgiveness, and how I can use the practice of mindfulness to stay calm and aware. Putting my thoughts in a positive space relieves my mind and relaxes my body. Things that I love to do—like create—lower cortisol in the body. How I react to life's situations—how I engage with my own perceptions and responses—creates opportunities for healing.

Reading literature and poetry by James Baldwin or Dr. Angelou or Nikki Giovanni opens my mind up and lets me connect to a range of emotions in a useful way. When I get to the theater and see people expressing their creativity, absorbing the playwright's expression through the energetic movement and speech of the actors, it's like a tower is being built in my mind, with each person's talents contributing to this space within me. The more I expose myself to the arts, the more that tower keeps building.

My mental diet becomes part of my sense of who I am and contributes to my philosophy on life. It gives me ingredients to help me understand more and feel more. It's like all of these artists are contributing colors that I can use to create my own inner emotional painting of the world. Listening to Coltrane, to Stevie Wonder, Nina Simone, Lauryn Hill—it all gives me more colors to paint with. All this mental stimulation makes my imagination more vivid, and as I receive in my brain, my mind creates something to put back into the mix.

Creativity has allowed me to find out things about myself that I didn't know, things that I wouldn't say to myself, things I would never dare say to anybody else. Through my creative processes, not only am I able to say it, but I'll say it out loud, even on the stage.

Self-understanding and compassion are things that I am always working on. Music has allowed me to express matters that are in my subconscious, that I hadn't really found ways to talk about in public, that I couldn't find a way to express in other ways. Music helped me break through the struggle of communicating what I really felt and gave me the freedom to feel less alone. When you're a creator, you're giving the world parts of yourself that may not even be healed yet. You're giving other people light but sometimes you yourself may still be sitting in darkness. Sometimes I haven't processed something before it goes into art.

Creativity doesn't have to be just for the public. Sometimes you just create to create, for the pure spirit of it. When I'm freestyling, I feel like I'm connecting with something divine and I can just let it pass through me. It's something I do with my mind that takes me to another place. That's how it feels to me.

Listening to music makes people happy. Singing lowers cortisol. Engaging with art is good for your mental health.[1] When you write lyrics or poetry, or when you write in a journal, you're exercising the mind and releasing ideas, thoughts, and feelings that you might not even know you've been holding on to. Putting feelings into words creates a story and an understanding. It's a way to see yourself and hear yourself in a different way, almost like being in conversation with yourself. Writing in an expressive way helps you reflect on life, reduces tension in your muscles, and lowers blood pressure. It's good for your memory and your mood.[2]

According to Harvard University, when we listen to emotional music, we're activating and synchronizing the parts of our brains that relate to emotion. The motor system of your brain also gets invited to the party, which is why you can hear the beat.

Music activates almost all of the regions and networks of the brain, including pathways that relate to your happiness, your well-being, and your brain function.[3] These activations matter because your brain pathways need to be used in order to stay strong. Since the brain is efficient and doesn't want to waste energy, if you're not using those pathways, they degrade so the neurons can be applied to something else. When you turn up the music, when you play music yourself, all the lights go on.

Art brings down barriers and puts you in a space of responsiveness and connection. It's fruitful to create and it's momentous to be the receiver of creativity. I loved being in a play and I love going to see plays; I love creating music and I love going to hear music. It's all feeding my mind, helping me feel inspired, a positive loop.

That's what I love about exposure to creativity and the way it relates to my own creative nature. Art amplifies joy so that you can feel that warmth and that happiness. It illuminates darkness when you're feeling the shadows of the mind and helps you step into the light.

As it says in Philippians 4:8, "Whatever is true, whatever is noble, whatever is right, whatever is pure, whatever is lovely, whatever is admirable—if anything is excellent or praiseworthy—think about such things."

Even in the darkest times, it's the way you think about yourself and talk to yourself that will get you through. It's the gratitude and compassion that will carry you forward. It's feeding yourself on beauty and elevation that will leave you inspired.

When you start thinking about the good things, you can get to more good things. When you think about powerful things, you become powerful within yourself.

Seeking Peace in a Troubled World

This past year, while working on this book, I was in London, filming *Silo*. It rained constantly, and I was very aware of it. The gray sky, the clouds, the dampness in the air. I like the rain, but I found myself very aware of the lack of sunshine and how much I was missing that. When you're in the sun on a cool day, that warmth touches you, and your whole body can relax. The effect of the sun on your face when it's cold, you can't miss the feeling of the experience. The moment it rolls over your skin, you just know. Your whole body recognizes the power of that sunshine, and you can feel what a difference it makes.

This was something I thought about a lot when I was in London. While I was over there, I realized one day that I felt a peace in my body that hadn't been there. This unfamiliar looseness in my body, I didn't understand it initially. I thought that it was because I was doing this project that I really loved. I was excited about playing this character, so I thought it was that. Then I thought, *Maybe London is just so dope, and it's because I'm getting to see all these plays and just hear good music.*

It took a while for me to understand that it was because I wasn't feeling like my body was a threat to this society, and I wasn't feeling threatened by this culture. Because my experience as a Black man was so different than what I was used to at home.

The day I figured it out, I was walking out of the hotel I was staying in, and the doorman, a guy named Fareed, cautioned me to hang back.

"Don't go down there," he said to me. "It's not safe."

He didn't want me heading down to Piccadilly Circus because there was a man with a gun.

I said, "What do you mean?"

"I don't know what's going on. We don't have guns like that out here."

I looked at him, as if to say, *Are you serious?*

He said it again. "We don't have guns like that out here."

That was when I started to notice that the police officers in London don't carry guns, and I realized just why my body had been feeling more relaxed, and why my shoulders felt looser, my mind was freer, my posture was better. It took Fareed saying it out loud for it all to come together for me.

No guns. It took something off my body that I had become accustomed to carrying around back home. I felt this space of relaxation in myself the whole time I was over there, and this was the reason. *No guns.* All I could think was, *Wow.* So many thoughts rose up and fit together. How Nina Simone moved out of the States. Why James Baldwin saw fit to leave. As Black people, the way we exist in the world, it's really something to suddenly feel a sense that you've let go of that tension that's always around you. Living with the threat of violence, with the constant knowledge of external dangers, it impacts the body on so many levels, and it impacts the mind, the heart, the soul.

Some places are a lot less threatening to your physical body. That's just how it is. There's still racism: they might say something to you, they might not give you the job, they might stereotype you. That doesn't feel good, but it's not the same as knowing that someone can just up and shoot you.

When I land back home in the States, the first person I see is holding a gun.

That's why I want to talk about how violence can affect the body and how it affects the mind, and how we need to do our best to try to find those things that we can use to overcome. My mother's no scientist, but she always told me, quit stressing because it causes disease. Turns out she knows what the researchers are just figuring out and writing papers on. Mental stress, emotional stress, affects the body and makes it harder for the body to fight illness.

The environment we are in becomes a part of us. Feeling warm, feeling safe, feeling protected does something to you. The opposite is also true. Feeling threatened, feeling frightened, feeling at risk, that does something to you, too. Those feelings change how our bodies feel. The shoulders tense up. The jaw locks. The brain is on high alert, so is the body. It's in your back, your arms, your neck. And it goes deeper too, into your nervous system, into your breathing, all the way down into your cells.

I talked with Dr. Tracey about how to care for my mind so that I can feel my best, be at my best, be my most creative self.

"It's like a garden," she said, about the mind. "If you want your plants to grow, you're going to need some sun."

She explained that the mind creates the environment that the body lives in because there's a relationship between your brain, your spine, your hormones, and your immune system.

"If we're going to talk about healing, then we have to talk about stress. That has to be a part of the conversation," she said. "There are two types of reactions in the body: stress response and relaxation response. The relaxation response is responsible for healing."

She says a lot of people are concerned about their physical aspects because they're easier to address than the mind, because as she says, "People don't often like to think about what's going on in their head." But what exists in our minds is made real in the body. We talked about the idea of mind over matter, and she explained that our mental energy actually is converted into matter.

The relaxation response is elicited from a body that is not on guard for danger. Imagine the feeling of getting a massage, or taking a nap in the sunshine under a tree. You feel warm and soft and at peace. In those moments, as when you're exercising, hanging out with loved ones, laughing, listening to music, your body is releasing hormones like dopamine, serotonin, endorphins, and oxytocin. This relaxation response can lead to your muscles relaxing, better digestion as blood flow shifts back to the gut, better sleep, and clearer thoughts. Peaceful thoughts and experiences lead to peaceful physical responses.

In contrast, when you feel threatened, it sets up a different kind of hormone download. When someone cuts you off while you're driving, you're stuck in a long line, you're treated in a way you don't appreciate—cortisol, epinephrine, and adrenaline are released, energizing you as this stress response ricochets through your body. A fight or flight response can be useful in a moment of crisis. But when you continually operate defensively, when all of life is a crisis situation, the result is inflammation and illness in the body.

We're always saying, *That stresses me out.* That stress isn't just of the moment. It's bigger than that. It sticks around. It messes with your whole body's functions for a long time. When you're feeling that stress all of the time, you can forget how unnatural it is, how unhealthy it is. But it's there with you, like a shadow, and over the years, if you're always having that constant vigilance, that all-the-time worry, it costs you. The research is out there if you want to read more about it. Our bodies carry the proof: racism and discrimination causes anxiety, depression, PTSD. It raises levels of diabetes. Raises blood pressure. Black men are more likely to die of heart attacks than white men. Black Americans get dementia twice as much as white Americans do. Black women are three to four times more likely than white women to have complications while giving birth or to die in childbirth.

To change these outcomes, the system has to change. Until that happens, we have to do whatever we can to take care of our bodies and improve our own health.

Knowing all of this, I believe that each move we do to take care of ourselves is a holy act and a revolutionary action. Our self-love is a shield we carry while we're out there doing the work to take care of our loved ones and working for change for all of those who are caught in this system of hurt. Everything you can do to take good and loving care of yourself matters even more when the world is not set up to give you the warm sun of love that you deserve, that you need to thrive. You've got to speak in the positive. You've got to speak into the light.

The world can be that agitator sometimes. The world can also exist as a reminder of how connected we are to something greater. All of us, the plants and the animals, too.

I was walking in a park in London, and there were these beautiful red flowers they call fire lilies. These flowers exist as a reminder of a higher plane. Even plants have relationships. There are ants and plants that need each other to survive. Even the trees talk to each other and share what they need to grow and live. We're all connected. We don't exist without one another. Nature is so amazing. The sun can warm us when we're cold, and it also makes the flowers grow. So does the rain. This is a beautiful world.

I am committed to learning how to access that and apply that and make it manifest while I'm in this dimension. The more we all connect to that more beautiful space, to that higher plane, to the spirit within us, the more that worldly tension eases. The more we protect our minds and our bodies, the more we can feel our power and use it for good and for glory.

Brighter Days

The barbershop is a place where as men we get to sit down and break bread and talk shit and build among one another. I've had some very meaningful talks about life with my barber and the same with my therapist. My time in therapy has shown me that the way I feel in situations and relationships comes from my perceptions as much as from what may be happening objectively. The way we perceive begins when we are children. Part of what therapy does is like changing the prescription of your emotional glasses to make sure that what you see in front of you is clear and true and not just a projection of your past experiences.

My path to therapy started with a broken heart. I was so sad, so hurt, just floating through life, unable to be truly present because I was struggling to understand that life had changed and shifted. I kept thinking, *But this is the person I'm supposed to love.*

God was saying, "I need you over here."

I was like, "Wait, wait. My heart is here."

I remember walking down the block with my cousin Ajile, God bless his soul. He was encouraging me, saying, "You're going to be okay."

His mother, my aunt Mattie, was talking with me late nights.

I was talking with my acting coach about what I was feeling, and she said, "You need to see a therapist. I know somebody who would be really good for you."

This was one of the hardest times in my life. Yet when I look back, I can appreciate that the pain is what started my quest for self-belief.

My acting coach introduced me to Susan Shilling, a social worker who counsels artists and creative people. Susan is very mindful about meeting people where they're at. She started her practice to help people, and along the way, she realized that part of her path was to become strong and whole herself so that she could support others. That's a perspective that I really respect.

My sessions with her are not long. They last for about forty-five minutes to an hour. She asks a lot of questions about what my life has been like, what I've experienced, about the parts that I feel have worked really well for me, and the parts that have not worked so well.

For this book, we talked about what therapy can give to a person.

"As human beings, we have storylines of things that have happened to us, and those experiences have shaped how we see things," she said. "The mind is a very powerful projector. We're putting our understanding of something, our fantasies, our desires, the information we're gathering, out onto something. How we interpret that in relation to ourselves is how we're going to feel."

According to her, within all of us "there's an underground river that has all of the information. It's the primordial soup of when we came into consciousness." Through therapy, we can get to know what's underneath. By examining my consciousness, I can work to keep my old experiences from creating a story in the present that isn't actually present and alive within a current relationship.

That's one of the fundamental benefits of therapy. You can get to know more about why you do what you do. You can see how your perceptions were shaped, and you can get tools to do something different. "If you have the will and the interest to do that work," said Susan, "when you do that work, there are gains that make you want to do more work. That's how we move as human beings." With a clearer perception, you can begin to make different choices instead of compulsively doing the same thing again and again, which just gets you to the same place over and over.

"A lot of us go through life trying to redecorate the house without working at the foundation of it," is how she explained it. "We'll put new carpets, we'll paint, we'll put new wallpaper, but when you start to go down deep, and go to the deeper level of the foundations, you might see that there's rotting or black mold or something that really needs some work, and we become afraid. That's normal.

"We become afraid that deep down inside, there are things that we've done that we feel bad about, that we have blocked and not dealt with, and we hold ourselves accountable in a way that's not helpful. To have empathy, forgiveness, compassion for yourself, you have to know what you're carrying around and what your house is built on. From there, once you start to feel that compassion, you can reach your inner child that has been trapped and traumatized. That's part of the therapeutic process. It takes someone very brave to want to go digging."

My experiences with therapy have helped me piece together the parts of my story from the past that were clouding my judgment in the present time. In my memoir *Let Love Have the Last Word*, I wrote about my experience being molested as a child by an older boy that I considered to be a friend. He was someone that I trusted, that my family trusted. I didn't understand what had happened, and I didn't process it at the time. I just knew that it didn't feel right to me and that a person I loved had done something to me that was a violation. I dealt with it by pushing it deep down inside of me. I didn't tell anybody. I didn't share it with my mother. I took it with me on my emotional journey, and I never examined how it might be affecting me until I went to therapy.

Now I have more insight into my own patterning, and I can pause in a confusing moment in a relationship situation and think to myself, *Is what I'm feeling really about me and this person? Or is it me dealing with old stuff and projecting it?*

Another aspect of my pain that has been revealed to me comes from my family relationships. Deep within me, my young self exists—a little Rashid who felt abandoned by his father. This hurt remained as pain and insecurity; this young part of me needed to be reassured and cared for and heard. He needed to be reminded that he's worthy, that he's worth it, that he's unconditionally loved. What therapy taught me was that I needed to tend to and care for that young version of myself so that his fears wouldn't keep defining me as an adult.

My relationship with my father was part of it. So is my relationship with my mother. The most love I have ever gotten was from my mother. It was just the two of us and, sometimes, my grandmother. The mother-son connection is already something. When you've got a single mom, and it's just you, you're everything to each other. They work, they sacrifice, and they give you what you are, and you feel that love strongly. When somebody else enters that family picture, it's a big shift.

I was eight years old when my mother remarried, and I had so many feelings around it. But I was too young to fully understand and process what it meant to me and what it meant for me. My lingering emotions from that era showed up later in my life as insecurities because of the discomfort I experienced back then. I wasn't able to communicate my feelings, and neither of us had the awareness to talk about it openly. Nobody sat me down to explain that I could never be replaced, that even though there would be another person in our home, I would always be her son. It was only through therapy that I was able to identify that some of my insecurities were rooted in this life event.

Because I wasn't living with my father, I was able to imagine him as a superhero. I didn't spend that much time with him, so who he was to me was an invention of my own imagination and desire. Susan's work with me in this regard has been so enlightening and life-changing because I can see that I'm a work in progress, and I can identify more readily when I'm bringing what eight-year-old Rashid felt to my adult relationships.

That's something I couldn't get from sharing my feelings about my broken heart with my friends, with my aunt, with my cousin. I needed the perspective of a professional who had a balanced, insightful view, who could share with me what they saw from the outside looking in.

"With a therapist, or with any other teacher, you want to feel seen and known in a deep way so that you can build trust," she told me when we talked about the value of therapy. "It's just really important to find somebody that you feel safe and connected with."

Susan helps me get to that place of telling myself that I'm deserving, that I'm worthy, that I have a part of me that needs to be nurtured and treated with love and let out into the light.

"When you've had an experience when you were younger, whatever that experience was, it's frozen in time. That part of yourself, your child, isn't aware that you've grown up," Susan said. "It's early experiences that have formed our understanding of who we are. When we're traumatized, we go into fight and flight. Fight and flight for children has to do with enormous arguments of their parents, violence, abandonment, things that happen early on."

Susan has helped me see the way all the things I've been carrying can affect the relationships that I'm in, how I want to feel that love, and I've also been scared to truly commit. I have had to work through those things, and she's been really supportive throughout that process.

As I've learned, if you don't take the time to acknowledge, you're not only living with it, you're still living in it. Susan and I have talked about how trauma in our younger years can lead to substance abuse. Like Susan said, "If you were raised in an abusive situation, and you have imprinted on that—this is what love looks like—then as you develop as a young person, you are going to seek out negative circumstances, unfortunately. In teenagers it becomes very dramatic and it can become self-harm; it can become lots of abuses—of drugs and alcohol, abusive relationships."

That's the cost of unnamed pain. My family has a history with alcoholism, which runs in so many people's families. My dad struggled with addiction, my uncle had his own challenges, and so have a lot of my heroes.

When I was younger, I was always out for a good time. I'm still someone who enjoys my life, but I'm more measured about how I approach drinking. One evening, I was at a dinner with my castmates from *Between Riverside and Crazy*, the Broadway play, and we were all enjoying ourselves. During the meal, I drank too much, and I felt it strongly the next day when I woke up with a hangover that depleted all my natural energy. I spent that day with my castmates, too, and I wasn't myself. I was quiet, hanging back. They were able to observe it because they were used to me being much livelier and more engaged.

That was when I said to myself, *Man, this isn't good for my body*, and I resolved to do it differently next time. I'd had too much fun, but it didn't mean the journey was over. Next time, I would be more thoughtful about my actions.

I've talked a lot about this with my trainer, Yancy, who has been through a lot of things himself. His journey to sobriety inspired him to become an addiction recovery coach and a meditation teacher as well as a trainer and life coach. "The whole fight to get clean and sober was a huge part of my journey," he said.

He got clean at age twenty-six, more than two decades ago, and he's been sober ever since. As he puts it, he has experienced "mental and spiritual well-being and happiness and joy that I had never had."

When it comes to drugs and alcohol, what Yancy tells people is that you can always do less. "You can have two drinks this week if you normally have five," he said. "You can certainly make progress in that regard. You can take an entire month off of drinking. When people take an entire thirty days off of drinking, you might go back to drinking after the thirty days, but your entire relationship with it is different. It gives you a space to get clarity."

"If you have a problem, as hard as it may be," said Yancy, "I think the most important thing is to go without, at least for a certain period of time. Space is best. If you're having a problem with addiction, that's where professional help is really important."

He strongly believes in the power of teamwork. "Inevitably, you're going to have your times, just being a human being, because of the ups and downs of life, you're going to have a tough time," he said. "If you have somebody that you've been working with the entire time, you're going to lean on each other. There's no way both of you guys are going to be weak at the same time. One is always going to be strong."

As Susan put it, "We need teachers. We've always had teachers, this is how we learn as human beings, it's how we are set up. Having a therapist, or having a priest, having a monk, somebody who is on a spiritual path who is trained in some way or another, all of that is essential for a deeper level of work."

Before therapy, I just kept moving forward, not realizing everything I was bringing forward with me. Now I can acknowledge what happened, how I reacted, what I pushed down deep inside me, and how I have been shaped by all of that. Because I've gotten a chance to explore my own darkness with the support of a professional, I have the tools to step back and consider my situations with clearer eyes, which helps me step out of the darkness into the light.

If there's anything you need to process, therapy can help you get to know yourself and express yourself more openly. It's like opening a window in a closed-up room and letting the sun and the breeze wash through.

Centering

Susan and I speak often about the idea of centering. Centering comes from meditation, physical exercise, eating right. All of these things center our nervous system, and when our nervous system is centered and our body is fueled and our mind is at ease, we then have a certain platform for creativity to expand. That's when we're at our most able and most competent.

"Think of athletes or dancers or yoga practitioners or even a flamingo," she said. "There is a center line that runs through the core of who they are physically, and from that part, when they lean over, they're not going to fall over because there is a center. A tall oak tree has deep roots into the ground, its trunk is firm. When the winds come, when the storm comes, the branches bend and everything is in motion. The trunk never moves. That's, in essence, what we're thinking about when we're thinking about how to hold ourselves in terms of perception."

These days, this feeling of comparison, of being looked at or talked about is even more pervasive because of social media. I was talking about it with Susan in a conversation about how that affects people's sense of who they are and who they feel they should be.

"It gives a sense of feeling less than," she said. "If the imbalance is on the outside, then it's about how long our legs are, or what kind of clothes we're wearing, or how nice the brand we're carrying is. If it's all based on the superficial, there isn't a balance of the whole person.

"The whole person comes from feeling good in yourself. What is your experience? Not what you should be; how is that person looking at you; what do you think that person is thinking of you. It's how are you feeling in this moment."

It makes me think about when I moved to New York, and I was developing my own personal style. I had these crochet pants that I liked to wear, this artsy stuff that was the culmination of me being who I am and being the individual that I was striving to be and just seeking out my own uniqueness. I got some reactions for those pants. People were talking about me, but I was okay with it, because so what? This is who I am. This is what I want to wear. This is what I choose to wear to show my individualism.

What bolstered me was also how I'd grown up because I was accustomed to being teased by my friends. I was used to the feeling of being made fun of around physical attributes. Having received that early on from a place of affection helped me build up that armor. The world wasn't doing it with love, to be sure, but I had already built up that self-love and confidence within myself. I had that acceptance of myself, so the comments fell away from me without touching me.

Besides, I wasn't getting dressed for external approval. I was and am dressing for myself. Clothes are part of expression, inspiration, creativity. There are influences and there is inspiration, but it's got to be for you.

To this day, the way I filter other people's reactions is smoother and easier when I'm centered in myself. When I'm calm and grounded, I can remember that everybody's going through something. I'm human; it can be a challenge not to take things personally when people are callous or unthinking. It helps to stay grounded in my own intentions, my own self, and when I am, I can understand that whomever I'm dealing with is emanating from their experience. Understanding that is so important.

Whatever they're going through when they lash out might be a really difficult situation. The more care I have for myself, the more centered I am, the more I can recognize their individuality and suffering and take a moment to consider what they might be going through.

The question is, how do we ground ourselves when we have so much coming at us? The first step in getting clarity mentally comes from the physical. Susan loves the twelve step programs that have an expression called HALT. It's about not getting too Hungry, Angry, Lonely, or Tired—because all of those experiences throw us into depletion, and we can't respond well when our nervous system is flooded.

"When you're feeling overwhelmed, when you are tired, when you are overstimulated, if you're in New York City, Chicago, busy streets, you will hear sounds and sirens and crashing and garbage cans, in a way that you will not hear them when you're not overwhelmed," said Susan. "Perception is mindfulness and grounding. This is where the mind and the body come together."

When I'm really centered and feeling good about who I am, it's harder to be angry and doubtful. It's harder to spew things out that don't need to be given to another individual.

Being centered allows you to realize that they may not be doing what you want them to do, but they're doing what they can because that's who they are at that moment, and it isn't all about you. It allows me to remember that I've got to meet people where they are. The more I remember that, the less their outbursts feel like they are about me.

"Compassion is everything," said Susan. "It starts with ourselves. Compassion is the softening of all the feelings that we have internalized, all of the anger, all of the not being enough. You really can't have compassion for someone else until you have compassion and forgiveness for yourself."

When you've been caring for yourself, when you're feeling good, when you're centered, you can go out in the world with enough love for self to be selfless with someone else.

That's grounding. That's understanding. That's being centered.

Leave the Bad Takes Behind

In 2010 I played in the NBA All-Star Celebrity Game in Dallas. I had been through extensive training with one of the Nets shooting trainers, who worked with me for hours on form, balance, patience, and control—all the things needed to make a really good athlete. I'm a solid basketball player, and I was feeling good about the game. Having been through extensive training, I knew that I was ready.

It was a dream to be able to run around on the court with actual NBA stars, but when it came down to it, I wasn't performing at the level that I normally would. It's funny because onstage, or in front of the cameras, I can feel relaxed. But I got on that basketball court and it wasn't the same; I didn't have that sense of ease. I think that just had to do with me not feeling comfortable under all those lights in the same way I do when I'm acting. I remember seeing Dwyane Wade, who perceived how disappointed I was that I didn't get MVP.

"Man," I said, "I just kept missing shots."

He was very supportive and told me that in the league, if you hit half of your shots, that's excellent because you're guaranteed to miss shots.

"You just got to have a short memory," he said. "That shot is what it was. It's done. You go on to the next play."

I understood what he meant. If you want to succeed on the next one, you have to believe that it's going to go in, no matter what happened the moment prior. When you miss, you have to try again, and you have to have that belief in self.

Ten years after that conversation with Dwyane, in 2020, I played in the All-Star Celebrity Game again, this time in Chicago. I had done my training, worked so hard to get myself tight for that game. One of my friends plays for the Portland Trailblazers, and he set it up so that I could train. Between being at home, my love for basketball, honoring all of that at once in this game, it was special. I was up and down the courts, working with the ball, working all the angles, getting myself in tune so I could show up and deliver my best. And I did. I got MVP this time, ten years after the last game.

That All Star weekend was special in so many ways. I got to judge the dunk contest alongside Chadwick Boseman. I didn't know that he was sick, and he ended up passing that summer, God bless his soul. I also got to do some spoken word that honored Kobe in a theater intro piece we created that focused on Chicago basketball, and I got to honor Kobe within the piece. That was a beautiful experience.

That's what I'm remembering now. That's what's sticking with me.

Leave the bad takes behind. Remember the shots that go in. I've taken what Dwyane said that evening with me, and I think of it often.

When I'm working to deliver my lines the way the director wants it to be, I'm always trying to give the take what it needs, but I'm not always delivering it the way I want to. Those times when it just isn't happening, I have to say to myself, *You've done everything you can do. You're giving your all. Leave the bad takes behind.*

Challenging yourself is healthy, and it is also damn hard. Making changes is so good for you, and it's damn hard. That's okay. Sometimes, we slide back into old habits. Falling away from the goal doesn't change the goal. The vision is still there. If you don't follow through on it at certain moments, that doesn't mean that it's over. It's a journey full of lessons to be learned. It's a path you're walking. When I'm filming, if there's one bad take, I don't just assume that every take that follows will be bad. I have to get it together and try again for the next one, and the next one, until it's right.

Sometimes even when you're like, *Okay, that take was bad*, you can still come in with the new energy so the next take will be better. If you're giving it your all, that's something to be proud of, too, even if it doesn't turn out the way you wanted it to. It's true in art and it's true in sports and it's true in how we eat, and in everything else that you do.

If you have a bad take, leave it behind. That take is gone now. Did it yesterday? It doesn't mean you have to do that again today. Did it today? It doesn't mean you have to do it again tomorrow. Focus on the next moment you have, on the next hour you have, on the next day you have. The scenes you see in a movie, the ones that compel you, the ones that you remember—you aren't seeing the bad takes. You're only seeing the one that worked.

Those are the moments we have to hold onto. As long as we are alive, we have a chance to make it right, to do better the next time. For the bad takes, you've got to have a short memory. For the good takes, carry that pride with you.

Be Transformed by the Renewal of Your Mind

Acting on a stage has a rhythm. It's not like performing music onstage; it's not like acting in a movie. Being in my first play, *Between*

Riverside and Crazy, brought a whole other kind of energy for me. Going through that process of acting, I was striving to find a rhythm, to see what the rhythm of acting is, the rhythm of the play, the rhythm of the language. It wasn't easy.

I love acting. I loved being on Broadway for the first time. It was a different path, but part of the same journey. I did it because I love acting and I feel a purpose in acting like I do with music. I have to work hard on my craft because acting takes a lot out of you, especially on a stage, but the goal is still the same. To give, to deliver, and to inspire; to bring people closer to themselves and their higher selves. Sometimes art is a reflection of truth that needs to be put out there so you can see yourself in it. It can be hard to get those rhythms, especially within a new thing, but it can also develop you in ways that you don't even know you're going to be developed.

There's an expectation around how I perform that comes from within me. That's why I work so hard on preparing: because the preparation allows me to be present. That's when I can let go and follow my intentions, and if something unexpected happens, I can adjust and respond because I've prepared. I've equipped myself to be present.

In this play, I was stepping into the consciousness of a character that was formerly incarcerated, on drugs, a character who wasn't at the best place in his life, and I had to bring the humanity to that person and allow him to be a full human being. I believe actors can inspire, heal, bring humanity to people because somebody else watching may be less judgmental if their uncle or their cousin is in that position.

When I was working on the play, it tested me physically, mentally, emotionally. I wanted to do well, and I felt that pressures of it being my first Broadway play. People would tell me that I had to focus because of the reviews . . . I wasn't thinking about the reviews. I was thinking about what I could do to bring my best. I do have all these methods and resources and practices to help me deal with that pressure. That included eating the foods that would give me the best energy, and my morning prayer, and reading the scripture. It included my workouts and everything I do to prepare for each show.

There are some things you can practice. That doesn't mean you won't feel any nervousness, but it just releases some of it. With that release, as the pressure eases, you can start to see that feeling as excitement and joy. Instead of saying, "I'm pressured," you can look at it more from a joyful perspective like, "I'm excited."

When people say, "You nervous?" I'll say, "Yes, I'm nervous, but this feels good. I care about this." Sometimes I'm happy when I sense my own nerves because it shows me that I really care. Being nervous is a way of feeling excited.

In order to tap into the excitement underneath it all, I have to really make sure I am eating clean and getting my workouts and trying to get enough sleep. It isn't just the pressure. It's the body needing that support, because when you go to emotional places as an actor, your body doesn't know that you're just acting. If your character is in pain, you have to feel that pain to get it across to the audience, and your body feels it, it experiences that pain night after night. You know that it's a play, but if you're conveying suffering, your body is suffering.

It made me think about those people who aren't acting, who are in pain every day, the pain of life, or illness, or worrying about how they're going to survive the situations they're in. You've got to do things to balance it out to combat that. "Be transformed by the renewal of your mind," the Bible says in Romans 12:2. If you're going to a stressful place every day, living that busy life, you've got to do things to feel better in body and mind.

I had a day where I was tapped into the pressure instead of the joy because I was stressing out about what the director wanted me to do. My reaction was that what he wanted was not the character. It was opposite of who I felt that this character was, and I wondered, *Am I going to deliver with this at the level that I want to?*

That night, working on that scene for the play, feeling down on myself, like nothing was going right for me, I realized that I needed to step back and take a break. Instead of being my best, all that was coming out of me was confusion and chaos, and I needed to leave that take behind.

I got some tickets to a basketball game at Madison Square Garden. Once I got my feet on the floor, just in looking around at the crowd, the athletes, the game I love, I felt good and right.

I came out of it feeling fresher and happier. The issues weren't resolved, but I had a new perspective, which allowed me to approach the situation in a new way.

Putting in the work matters. So does resting easy. That's something I've had to learn because when you're out there trying to make it, you make the hustle the focus. You start to feel that if you let go for a moment, you might not be able to grab hold again, but it's the opposite. You've got to give yourself those moments of pure downtime in order to get back up again and do your best.

That's something I've learned from people who are at the top of their game, who create at the highest levels because they also make space for peace and for quiet moments.

I remember being at a birthday dinner celebration for Nas in New York with Jay-Z and the brilliant businessman Steve Stoute, tasting good wines, and we were talking. Steve Stoute was giving us a lot, giving each of us a lot. We were talking about life, about getting older, about how we love on our people and love on ourselves.

Our conversation turned to our favorite spaces for vacation and relaxation, and Jay said to me, "What are you going to do for yourself?"

I laughed and said, "I don't take vacations!"

He looked at me straight and asked, "What are you talking about? What do you mean you don't take vacations?"

I thought I was being funny, saying that I didn't have time for vacations because I was always working, as if that was a positive and mighty aspect of being. He wasn't having it because he saw it in a whole other light. It was one of those things that made me pause because this is a man who is extremely successful, who recognizes the value in having that balance, of going to just relax your mind, take care of self, and renew.

It was enlightening for me to take that in and think, *I need to start doing this.*

Because of that, I started to make an effort to take that space for myself, where nobody is asking me for anything, where I have time to reflect and renew myself. It may be only a few days, like going to a resort where I can get massages and be in the desert. I had a birthday and decided to go to Turks and Caicos, and it was so healing to have those times to just do those nice things.

When it's the moment of creation, you have to be there with

your whole self. That's being present. You also have to step away from the work at times. That doesn't mean that you need to get on a plane in order to feel that peace. Doing nothing is still doing something when that is what's needed. Those days where you allow yourself to do nothing, to just be, can be the most valuable days of life, when you don't have any scheduled work, any obligations, and you just do exactly what you feel like doing. You can rest your body by laying down. You can watch a game. Take a walk. Listen to some music, or play some music if that's what you do.

There is divinity in rest. Even God rested! I am grateful to have been reminded that it's a good thing to give myself peace of time while I'm looking for peace of mind. We were created to create, but we were also meant to rest. Being whole, well, and rested is our divine inheritance.

Taking It Back to the Community

As I was working on this section of the book, I went in Chicago to celebrate the election of Mayor Brandon Johnson. What drew me to this individual, the reason I threw my energy into supporting his campaign, was a conversation we had about mental health support. One of the things that I really appreciated and valued was that his approach to stopping violence was to provide jobs and to give mental health support, preventing people from getting to those places of violence.

Not many leaders have come with that type of idea, and we have definitely not heard them talk about mental health like that in Chicago. This is a young Black man that's talking about that, and it's good for us to hear, good for us to know, and good for us for it to be implemented because it really can be effective in preventing people from falling into a lifestyle of crime and violence. I was drawn to supporting him because I'm interested in the practical things that people can use in their lives. We need leaders who want to bring that to the people.

The roots of violence begin in youth, and the more we support young people with help—before these issues have time and space to become actions that lead to more harmful actions—the healthier these individuals will be, the healthier our neighborhoods will be, the healthier our cities will be. Kids who are growing up within violence, when they grow up and express themselves in violent ways—it's because they haven't experienced compassion, and they don't have compassion for themselves, and so how are they going to have compassion for others? Anyone who loves themselves, who truly has compassion, cannot go out and hurt another person. If you have been taught to have compassion for yourself, then you will have the capacity to have compassion for others. Like Susan said, "When we are nurtured, at any age, by any type of thing, we tend to thrive because we're set up to evolve."

I know there's a long way to go, and I salute all of the people out there doing the work, dedicating their whole lives to working with people who are incarcerated, to working with children and with kids in the foster care system. I just want to be a part of the work, and that includes working on self. Because of my work on self, I've reached the level in my life, the point in my life, where the activity and actions of actualizing things brings so much reward to me. When I can participate in things that help people work, have jobs, change their lives—that is meaningful to me. To go visit human beings in prison and to listen to them and talk to them. To know that someone came out of prison and was able to get work at a tech company. To see bills passed that support juveniles in California, where they are no longer sentenced to life without parole, that really hit me in my soul.

There are ideas and paths of consciousness that I didn't have access to when I was growing up. Though music, I've been blessed with the path and the opportunities to see and experience things that have helped me to learn myself. Because of my work, I have traveled to different places, and I've met individuals with ideas that have shaped me in positive ways. The beautiful thing is that I have gotten to pick the pieces that really work for me, that help me to be the best person I can be. On my journey, I have been finding joy within myself and love for myself that is so strong and so overwhelming that I can share it with others. I've been able to get a lot of inspiration and love and good energy, and now, I want to give that back to people. I have joy when I see others achieving their dreams, becoming better human beings, and being better within themselves, loving themselves more, building their relationships with God and themselves. Just thinking about these ideas, doing this work, sharing it with others as much as I can: this is the most in tune with myself that I have ever felt in my life.

During the pandemic, I was giving my team as much support as I could on a personal level. I invited them to go to therapy, and people would reach out to me and say, "I want to go. Thank you. I'm dealing with stuff right now, this is really difficult."

We've always been a family, but going to those tougher places together was very emotional for me. To be able to offer that support and have it be received so fully made me feel like we were achieving success together in a different way. One of the guys who works with me reached out and said, "I've been going to therapy, and now I'm going to get married. This is the best I've felt . . . Therapy changed my life. You used to talk about it, and I didn't really understand what you were talking about. I'm dealing with stuff that I've never dealt with."

All of this leads to me operating at my highest level. What we give to ourselves, what we can share with others: that's what is important to me. That's how I measure success now.

I want to see people achieving evolution and growth, to see people become inspired to make decisions to be better in their lives. That's why I wrote this book. Because your joy is a part of my joy, and your happiness makes me happy. I want to rise, but I don't want to be on that mountaintop alone. I want you up there with me.

Aging and the Mind

In honor of Mother's Day, I took a trip down to Florida to visit my mother and my grandmother. That first afternoon, my mother and I were together, chilling and talking and enjoying some good quality time. The next day, we went over to see my grandmother at the home where she was living.

My grandmother is my heart. When I was young and my mother was working a lot, my grandmother would walk me to school. As she always tells it, I would ask her to walk on the other side of the block so that I could look like I was going to school by myself. I don't remember that; she holds that story for me, and I only know the details because she has shared it with me so many times.

The two of us have always had a very close relationship. Through the years, I would call her and ask her to pray for me because I was going out for an audition, was about to do a movie, or we were up for an audition, was about to do a movie, or we were up for an Oscar. For all of those times, full of eagerness and anticipation and hope, she was there. For the difficult times in my life, she was there, too.

At the time of this visit, she was ninety-five going on ninety-six. She'd had two strokes. She had shingles. She'd been dealing with a lot. The last time I had seen her, over Christmas, she knew who I was, and she had been really talking with me. But over the year before this visit, she hadn't been the same, as my mother shared with me. Before we went, my mother told me that she had been declining since I last saw her. I had to prepare myself to go and see her on this Mother's Day. I was praying for her mind now in her body because she was at her older age.

When we walked in, my grandmother was standing with other elderly people. She saw me and she said, "Hey, boo. You look good. Your shoes look good."

As we were sitting and talking together, her mind wasn't fully in our conversation. Some things that she talked about, I was not familiar with. It was obvious now that she didn't know either, as she kept shifting the topic to something that was happening somewhere else, at some other time. We just kept progressing, agreeing with her, and I began to realize that we were treating her like she was a child, just going along with whatever she suggested conversationally because her mind was occupying these various spaces.

After a while, we went out to get some air, and there were musicians performing and other activities happening around us at this facility for the elderly. She didn't want to be there, didn't want to be outside. I could tell that she was drifting out and that she didn't know who I was anymore. I felt it. My mother felt it.

When I was young, she knew more about me than I knew about myself. My mother prepared me for her decline, but I still wasn't ready for that feeling of my grandmother not knowing who I was.

When the memories of our elders slip away, we can take those stories they have shared and make them our stories, but we can't truly remember what they have forgotten. We can think back to what they have told us about their experiences, but we can't truly know what they saw when they were young and coming up. It is a loss, for them and for us.

We said our goodbyes so that she could rest, and we took our leave.

My mother believed that my grandmother's memory loss was related to the pandemic and to the time she'd spent stuck inside, just watching TV. In her younger years, my grandmother was so active. Between doing manicures and taking care of me and everything else she did, she was accustomed to a rich, full, engaging life. Being indoors in front of the TV, unable to see our family, kept her from exercising her mind in a healthy way. That was her opinion, and it resonated with me.

She knows how I think, and as we were leaving my grandmother's room, she made sure to say, "You know, when you get older, it might not be like this for you."

Some people make assumptions around age, expecting that you're going to get arthritis, you're going to have health issues, you're going to become very forgetful. My mother wanted me to understand that I may not become forgetful as an older person, and that I don't need to anticipate that when I am old, I won't be able to move or think. I really appreciated her expressing this to me as I was processing my grandmother's experience.

Not long after this visit, I had a talk with Dr. Tracey, who told me that my mother was right. We should not be anticipating dementia as a regular side effect of age because not everyone ages in the same way. Two people with the same birthday may have very different health outcomes as the years go by. That's because chronological age, which is based on your birth year, doesn't tell the whole story. How we age is more closely related to what we call our biological age, which is linked to the ways that our genes and lifestyle express themselves in our cells.

Dementia is not a fact of life, but according to the Alzheimer's Association, 55 percent of Black people believe that experiencing memory loss and cognitive decline will naturally occur as people age. This is not true. Dementia is a disease, and it is not a given that you will get a disease of dementia when you get older.[4] (To be clear, dementia is a blanket term for a decreased ability to remember things, to think, and to make decisions. The most prevalent kind of dementia is Alzheimer's disease.) With awareness and preventative care we can experience an old age that includes movement and mental acuity, if we are fortunate.

It's important for us to have insight and awareness about aging and the way our minds can be affected, especially within the Black community because researchers have found that Black Americans are two times as likely to get Alzheimer's or another kind of dementia. While they can't explain precisely why that is,[5] according to the CDC, it relates to heart disease, diabetes, and discrimination and adversity exposure. Estimates say that within the next thirty-five years, cases of dementia among Black Americans will increase four times from today's numbers.[6] This makes me sad, and it makes me angry.

Until the processes are in place to protect us, we have to protect ourselves however we can. I'm not here to put pressure on individuals for things that should be in effect in a much larger societal way, but in a world that isn't shielding us, we need our own armor, our own tools, our own know-how. It's not fair to put this responsibility on individuals. It really isn't. But until the system changes, while it changes, we have got to take care of our minds and bodies.

According to Dr. Tracey, there are doctors who specialize in aging and longevity, including within the alternative medicine or integrative medicine fields where people are proactively seeking to avoid certain kinds of illnesses. If you're healthy now, and you don't want to have Alzheimer's, don't want to have Parkinson's, don't want any form of dementia, there are ways to fortify your mind and body to reduce the risk.

Food, sleep, exercise, and mental stimulation are all ways to care for your brain. Dr. Tracey and I talked about the difference between the various fats in the food that we eat. The brain is composed of 60 percent fat, along with water, she said, continuing, "That's going to tell you right there that you're going to need some pretty healthy fats."

Trans fats, found in foods like donuts and fried chicken, are oxygenated and unhealthy for the body and brain. Those are the ones we want to avoid. Then there are the unsaturated healthy fats, found in foods like avocados, chia seeds, and flaxseeds, which support brain health.

"If you want the best out of your brain," she told me, "then you're going to have to feed it those things."

Your fitness comes into play here, too, because exercise isn't only about looking cut. Working out provides your brain with needed oxygen, keeping it vital and healthy.

Our brains can benefit from our choices during the day and at night because sleep is another aspect of brain health. When you're asleep, your brain recharges. The quality of your sleep affects how you feel the next day, and it has cumulative effects when it comes to the vitality of your mind.

Taking care of ourselves now shapes and affects who we become in our older years. That's what this taking care of yourself is about: the idea that if you are blessed to live into these older years, you can still be vibrant and moving around with vitality. I'm thinking of Cicely Tyson, whom I saw on Broadway doing a play called *The Trip to Bountiful* in her late eighties, just tearing it up, and of Rita Moreno. Staying at their level because of their artistry, using their minds, reciting lines, exercising the imagination.

The brain is a physical part of us. It's the seat of our intellectual selves. It's where our feelings originate from. It holds our memories and our stories and the details of our connections to other people. The more we train our minds as well as our bodies, the sharper we can remain. Learning a new language, playing a musical instrument, traveling, trying new things—that all plays into your mental acuity. The more you build these connections in your brain, the more your brain has pathways to rely on, even as some of them deteriorate naturally with age. That's another reason for prioritizing your mental diet, eating well, exercising the body, and getting that good sweet sleep in.

Caring for the mind supports you on so many levels, for today, tomorrow, and all the years that will follow.

The Muhammad Ali Theory

While I was filming *Smoking Aces*, Jamie Foxx reached out to me to say that he wanted me to do a song with him. Part of me wanted to keep all of myself focused on doing my best in this role, but he was hyping it up, telling me all about it, making promises, telling me that if we did this song, we'd go on Oprah's show and perform it for her. That was how confident he was in what he wanted to do. The song hadn't even been done yet, and in his mind, he already knew how it would go.

I had never done Oprah's show, but it was also Jamie Foxx asking, so he didn't really need to sell me on it. Because it was him, I said yes.

A month later he called me, telling me that we were going to do this song, which was about a man telling his pregnant wife how beautiful she was, on *The Oprah Winfrey Show*.

I was so excited! I got a new suit. I told my mother. I flew myself there, and I flew my barber there. I rode up to that lot so full of enthusiasm because I was going to be on Oprah. Being from Chicago—being from anywhere—this was a very big deal.

As I was waiting on set for Jamie to arrive, one of Oprah's executive producers came in and said, "Common, what are you doing here?"

This was one sign that something was not as I anticipated, but I told him that I was there to rehearse because we were doing this song.

Jamie's music director came in and said, "Common, what are you doing here?"

That was the next sign.

Upon Jamie's arrival, I learned that, in fact, we were not scheduled to perform that day. His plan was just to present it to Oprah on the spot as a surprise—however, it was actually possible that we wouldn't get to do it on the show.

All I could say was, "Really?"

While they were filming, I was in the green room, waiting and watching and wondering what I was doing there. I was so confused and frustrated. All I wanted was to get out of there and get some air.

I turned to my manager and said, "I've got to take a walk."

My manager said, "Don't leave."

I waited in the green room, watching Jamie interact with Oprah and observing his calm and his charm. In between segments, I heard him talking to her, mentioning me, working it out.

As they finished the segment, they called me out, and we performed the song with no rehearsal at all. Jamie did his part, and I did mine, and he called Oprah up in the middle of the song, and everyone there had a very good time. I was glad I had come, and I was glad I had stayed. The song didn't make the show, but it appeared as part of the aftershow.

Backstage, post-performance, Oprah showed us pictures of a home she was building in Santa Barbara. There was so much joy in what she was sharing with us. She was telling us how beautiful it was, explaining how it was going to be arranged, what she was going to build in the various areas. What struck me was how excited she was, how peaceful. There wasn't a moment where I felt like she was doing it to make us feel bad. She was coming from a place of love for what she was creating. Seeing those acres of land, I felt so inspired.

I was raised to feel like you shouldn't brag, as if there were something next level about being humble about your accomplishments. Yet I've always admired people that come in with the confidence, with the joy of their own accomplishments, the kind of pride that is about understanding your own self-worth. It's taken me time to understand the difference between bragging and putting yourself above other people, and just having confidence in yourself. When it's about your own understanding of the beauty of doing what you set out to do, not about needing to raise yourself up by knocking other people down, that's a beautiful thing.

That's the Muhammad Ali theory. "I am the greatest. I said that even before I knew I was," is a quote that is attributed to him. Is that bragging? Or is it setting yourself up to succeed? It seems dishonest to have to knock yourself down a few pegs just to satisfy other people who aren't out there trying their hardest and discovering what their best looks and feels like. It's okay to be your own hype man and hype woman. It's good to be your own champion. To know what you have done, what you are trying to do, what you are proud of doing, that's not bragging. That's confidence. I don't think anyone should be condescending. I do think we should have faith in who we are and love for who we are.

As a young Black kid, seeing Muhammad Ali, seeing someone who looked like me succeed in that way, made me realize that I could actually be something. I had never seen Ali box, not one match, but his words gave me everything. Muhammad Ali planted those seeds in me that made me feel like I belong, like I'm valued, I'm great, I'm special. I got something in me. I am beautiful. His confidence instilled that in me. Realizing that it is okay to live within that confidence and project it outward moved me. When it's done with love, confidence transfers from one person to the next.

I once did an interview with Muhammad Ali's wife, Lonnie

Ali, and she responded to something that I said with the words, "What you just said reminded me of Muhammad."

I said, "You're touching my spirit now."

I admired that man so much, his energy and what he brought to people, what he did for little Black boys and girls who needed to know that they meant something, that they were of value, and that they could be. He instilled hope and he exuded power. Ali was a light. He showed me that I could be a light. So did Dr. King and Dr. Angelou and Malcolm X.

If you love yourself, if you're proud of yourself, it creates a space for enthusiasm, for excitement, for other people to get into what you're doing and be happy to share what they themselves are doing. I walked into that performance with doubt, and I walked out of that day with a new idea about self-belief. I learned from Jamie's confidence in what he wanted to create, how he pulled us all together, how he arranged things so that it could flow in the way he imagined. He didn't worry. He didn't stress. He had faith in himself, in me, in everything turning out in a positive way. I learned from Oprah's contagious joy about this home she was creating. She was so happy about it, so happy to share it with us. I will never forget her glow, the way she just embraced it.

Bragging comes from doubt. Self-appreciation emanates from faith and confidence. That's what I want for myself, and what I want for you. Pride in yourself. Joy in whatever you are doing. Belief in what you are putting into the world, and acceptance that you are worthy of it.

We all deserve a mindset that is calibrated to rejoice in our blessings.

PART 4

THE
SOUL

" When I sing, I sing to try and bring Enlightenment. "

—KRS-One, "Breath Control"

A Spirit of Power and of Love

My first spiritual teacher was my mother. When I was growing up, she was adamant about me going to church and making sure that I said my prayers at night. Every Sunday, she would take me to church. That was our routine.

One Sunday morning when I was eight years old, we were on our way as usual to a church called Unity. We got there and it seemed like everyone else in Chicago had the same idea, like each one of us in that city had woken up and said, "Well, it's Sunday, let's go to Unity." That was how crowded it was. The church was so packed with people that there just wasn't any room for us. So many people had come to pray that morning that they were out of seats, so we had to think of somewhere else to go.

My mother's friend suggested we try a church called Trinity. As we went over there, as we walked into the Trinity United Church of Christ, my expectation was that it was going to be a Sunday like any other Sunday. But this day, God blessed me with a new feeling, a new realization about His power and His word.

Reverend Jeremiah Wright was in the pulpit. He started to preach, and I felt it. I felt the charge. I felt the energy of his message. I was electrified by what I was hearing and seeing around me. It was a celebration of God and of Black culture. I felt the power in myself, and it was a Godly power and it was a Black power. I didn't understand everything that he preached about, but I understood a lot, and more than that, I felt it. I could see how the other people were moved by what they were experiencing, and that moved me, too.

That was a moment for me in my understanding of what church could be like, of what this relationship with God could bring to you. I felt so grateful that morning that Unity didn't have a seat for us. Instead of doing what we had planned, we did what God planned for us, and what we discovered at Trinity was a call to glory for me that I have never forgotten.

Being in the pews in Trinity United Church, it was like God was speaking to me. I felt like I was learning God. I felt inspired by my Blackness. I was charged up by being in the presence of God. I've held that feeling close ever since.

God has been the source of the most beautiful and greatest relationship that I have known and ever will know. The more I build on that relationship, the more I take time to spend on that relationship, the more I feel closer to Him. That relationship makes me feel stronger, more compassionate, and more understanding. I have purpose and I have joy and I have inspiration.

The reason I continue to say relationship is because I'm not really a person who believes that religion is the only construct that gets you closer to God. I'm a person that grew up going to church, and people would call me a Christian. When I was twenty-one and read *Awakening the Buddha Within*, I didn't have to be Buddhist to understand that the practice of love is important. That's the same thing Jesus spoke about. I believe that people from different spiritual practices are in tune with God. I just chose the pathway of Jesus to reach my higher self and to communicate with God. If someone else is choosing something else, I don't knock that because that's their path to their higher being. I believe somebody that's studying Islam is close to God. That's their pathway to get to God. That's their relationship.

Religion has been developed by human beings as a path to God, and as they passed it on, those people passed their own ideals down within it, too. There may be things in religion that enhance you or give you more understanding; you have to decipher those things for yourself, and you have to use your own discernment to extract whatever doesn't resonate with you. It's the relationship with God that is the most valuable and cherished thing.

The more and more I build my relationship, I think about what that means. What does that mean for me in life? How do I apply that to my life and become the highest being that I'm supposed to be? That's the question. Not what is your relationship with the religion, but does it allow you to get closer to God? The way I see it, when it comes to spirituality and a relationship with a higher power, there's nothing that can come between you and that higher power, between you and the Source, the Creator of the heavens and Earth. Nothing comes in between that. There's a strength in knowing that it's your relationship with God that is most important.

I'm blessed to have been introduced to my soul when I was very young. It's why I've always talked to God, said my prayers, and acknowledged God in things. This connection allows me to see the Spirit all around me, to recognize that Spirit in myself and in others. The stronger that connection grows, the more I do my best to live in a way that is true to that.

Being at your best is honoring yourself, and it is honoring God.

Let the Morning Bring Me Word

This book was created with four pillars. It all leads to this space of the spiritual because wellness has the power to go deeper. When I talk about eating well, when I'm working out, I'm going to the deeper place of what that means in my life, and what I hope it can be for somebody else's life. Care of the body is spiritual because it clears the mind, and a clear mind can determine what the soul needs. Health of body and health of mind is a spirit thing. Success and activism also come from the spirit place, and so does music and creativity. It all comes from the spirit.

That's why I begin each morning in the same way. I thank God for the morning and I thank Him for the day.

No matter what day, no matter what happened yesterday, or what might be on my calendar for today. I can wake up with a strange feeling, but I'm still going to thank God for the day. I'm still going to say, thank you for this beautiful day. There have been weeks where uncomfortable events were taking place, situations that were tough, that had me down, but I still thanked God for the day to come.

"Thank you, God."

I say it because I mean it. Whatever is coming, I have gratitude within myself every morning. That's how I begin the day because I understand where I begin—with God. Where did my life begin? With God. What is the truest, purest connection that I've had in my whole life? With God. I go to that connection because it reminds me of who I am. As the church folks say, "Whose I am."

Thanking God reminds me what I'm capable of and what I've been gifted with. When you start looking at the qualities of God, you start realizing all the beautiful things that you are supposed to have, that you are destined to have, that were created for you.

When you open the day with the news, or with gossip, or with chatter about ugly things that may be happening in the world, that situates you in the negative. When you enter the spiritual realm in those early morning hours, you're in a space of calm, a realm of love, with no hatred and no jealousy or fear.

Those human emotions just fall off. They are removed and extracted from you. If you go in there with a pure heart, full of gratitude, seeking that connection, that's what you will receive. That realm is where you will find yourself existing. That's why I read scripture. I love the New Testament because it helps me remember why I'm here, and there are other parts of the Bible that move me in the same way.

I might read from Philippians 4:12–13, "I have learned the secret of being content in any and every situation, whether well fed or hungry, whether living in plenty or in want. I can do all this through him who gives me strength."

Or from John 15:16–17, "You did not choose me, but I chose you and appointed you so that you might go and bear fruit—fruit that will last—and so that whatever you ask in my name the Father will give you. This is my command: Love each other."

I might turn to Jeremiah 17:7–8 and meditate on the beauty of the lines, "But blessed is the one who trusts in the Lord, whose confidence is in him. They will be like a tree planted by the water that sends out its roots by the stream. It does not fear when heat comes; its leaves are always green. It has no worries in a year of drought and never fails to bear fruit."

I know that throughout my day, if I can stand on these words, lay back on these words, move forward on these words, and bring them into action, this day will be great.

After I do my reading, I do a meditation. I sit quietly at the side of the bed and consider my intentions. It's a practice that I've created for myself, woven from ideas about meditation that I have picked up from various people that I respect. It's my way to center myself, to create a calming space, to return to a spirit and a space of power.

It sets me up to create my own happiness, from the inside. There may be a day where it's raining and storming, and I might be wishing that it was a sunny, warm, beautiful day, but I don't control that. What I do control is my ability to realize that a rainy day is also a beautiful day. You can't determine what the weather will be, but you can work on your awareness, your acceptance, your ability to receive and transform. Even a rainy day is a great day when you're in that space of openness and acceptance.

As I get older, the things that I want for my life change. The music that I used to play will change. So will the music that I'm creating because we are always in a new place. Change is always with us. Through that, my practices are a constant. There was a time when they were choices, but they have grown to become integral parts of me. Some changes we don't control. The changes we create in our own lives are up to us.

My practices ground me, they focus me, they remind me who I am and how I want to move through my life. Change is always coming. Reading scripture is a constant. So is doing my meditation. The things I meditate on might change. The goals change, the visions change, the dreams change. Me taking time to myself at the beginning of the day to commune with myself remains consistent.

My scripture, my meditation, helps me to express my intentions clearly to myself. The way I eat, my commitment to bettering the body and the mind, it all takes me to that place where I can bring myself some joy and bring myself some happiness.

For me, the practice of wellness is one that leads me to my higher self. The higher self is the parts of one's being that are greater than the body and connected to the higher source of God. That is pure and true to the soul; that has an intention, in a way, about it; that is not only about self, even though it's the higher self. It's like the higher self has an ability to operate on several levels of our existence. When you are working from a place of understanding and compassion and kindness, it takes you being your higher self to do that. We have to take care of our human self to get to the higher self. If you're hungry and you're tired, it's harder to access. That's what you do these wellness practices for—to go through the process so you can get to the higher self.

It's hard for me to not take in the pain of the world. Of course, I feel it. I'm a human being with compassion. I care. My way of dealing with the tension of daily life, all the problems in this world, starts with me. That's why I'm doing the things, taking care of myself first, really having that God relationship and knowing that God is within me and within you.

Whatever spiritual practice you take, that's true for you, however you like to express it. The Buddha that's within you. The Spirit that is within you. I have the power of Christ. You have that within you, too. Psalms 82:6 says, "You are gods; you are all sons of the Most High." I believe that Christ is a spirit that exists within us. We are all connected to the creator of the heavens and Earth. Whatever you believe, you are connected to a higher power. It helps me to not get sucked into the world's worries because I know things exist on another plane. When we're on that higher plane, nobody can pull us down by arguing, by dragging us with their words.

There are a lot of challenges out there, so many things going on. It's tough. There are guns and there are wars. There's outward hatred and there's quiet sadness. There are earthquakes and there are hurricanes. Some people have said to me, "Man, well, if you believe in God, why did God let these things happen to people?" I will not just say that everything in the world is terrible. Some of these things are man doing it to man. We have dominion. We have power that we can exercise for good. It takes practice to remember that the world is also a wonderful place.

After I do my reading and my meditation, I drink water, take my supplements, and then I take my green juices down to the gym for my workout.

That's my time. From there, I'm ready to take on the day.

Life Is Breath, Breath Is Spirit

In Genesis 2:7, it says, "Then the Lord God formed a man from the dust of the ground and breathed into his nostrils the breath of life, and the man became a living being."

Breath is the beginning of spirit.

Dr. Tracey and I talked about the connection between spirituality and health. "Spirituality is the way of life. My way of life is the way I move, live, and breathe healthy," she said, pointing out that the word *spirituality* comes from a Latin word that means breath.

"For people, breath signifies life. When breath ceases, life ceases," she told me. "All living things breathe. Even cells respirate.

They breathe. We're an oxygen-based system, so all living things breathe so that life becomes breath. We all have this gift of life within us. The minute a baby is born, the first thing they do is to suck life. You start off with this gift."

Breath is spirituality. Every time Coltrane lifted that saxophone to his lips and blew into it, it was a measure of spirit. So are the words we use when we speak, rap, sing. KRS-One has a song called "Breath Control" in which he says, "I like clarity, so when you come here / Speak clear and concise."

It was so key as a rapper to not lose your breath because that's how you keep going. Breath control was one of the things that was celebrated if you were an MC or an artist. The biggest compliment we could pay was to say, "Man, that guy has breath control." All the best rappers, even if they didn't know it, they were using breath in their technique.

When I was working on my album *Resurrection*, I would go jogging and say my raps while I was running so that I would have control when I got into the studio. I continue to do that to this day, saying my rhymes while I'm on the bike or moving outside.

It's crucial for my acting, too. When I was doing the play, breath was so important. It made me realize how important breath is to everything I do. The attention to breath, the appreciation of it, the actual intention of taking a deep breath—I was working with a voice coach and the most important thing he told me was where to breathe from as I used my voice. That breath needed to come from all parts of my body in order to be effective. Not only from below my diaphragm. I needed to feel that breath in my toes, my knees, my shoulders, my whole body. To this day, I think about this.

When I was working on *Silo*, I was holding myself in a way that didn't feel as right or natural as I wanted for Sims, my character. I felt like I was moving my head too much while I was speaking, and I wasn't sure how to change it. I was in my body because I did exercises that would give me that body awareness, but I was still holding tension, and it was showing.

I asked my acting coach about this, and we talked to my vocal coach, who suggested that the way to shift that was to focus on the breath. The advice I got was to breathe, to use the breath, and not to tense up just because it's a tense scene.

He had me doing vocal exercises that began with taking deep breaths. When the acting feels grounded, it's because I'm centered in my breath, because the breath is coming from a place in my gut area, and because the thoughts are coming from that space of having breath. Only with that as a foundation can you really think at your best.

Dr. Tracey makes a similar connection. "The way we love, the way we think, the way we speak," she said. "Life is living through me by how I express that breath. My thoughts, my words, my choices are being made with my mouth, with the air that I breathe. The God in us is expressed by how we express ourselves."

I learned this lesson from Dr. Angelou as well, from her belief that every word we use matters. At Dr. Angelou's invitation, I went down to North Carolina to visit with her. We talked a lot and ate together, and even though we ate differently, she made sure I had what I needed, with her being the motherly figure, the grandmotherly figure. We just had a wonderful time, and I asked if she would be on my album project *The Dreamer/The Believer*. She agreed, and when you listen to the song "The Dreamer," you can hear her words.

Dare to let your dreams reach beyond you.
Know that history holds more than it seems.
We are here alive today because our ancestors dared to dream.

On that album, I was saying the word *nigger*, and when she heard it, she let me know that she was not happy with it. We had a conversation, and she told me what it meant to her. She explained that she put her voice on my album and that me using that word wasn't something that she wanted to endorse. I heard everything she was saying, and I made sure we took it off the next print because I respected what she was saying. When I'm in tune because I am practicing and building my relationship with God, it allows me to connect with others and to exchange the type of love that makes me better. She lived according to her beliefs, and she was clear with me where she stood. I received her ideas, and I behaved accordingly. That's spirituality, too.

My spirituality is a part of my wellness; my wellness is a part of my spirituality. To me, the pursuit of wellness is about the self-love that can lead me to my higher self. I think, *How can I love myself enough so that I can be myself and be happy and joyful in myself and be strong within myself and empowered and free to be myself?* Self-love is necessary for all of those things.

Every time you breathe in and out, you are expressing your connection to divinity. That's the root of self-care, the root of self-love, and a connection to God, the creator of the heavens and Earth that exists in all beings and that has been here since time began, and an infinite being whose qualities are love and joy and peace and understanding, hope and faith and creativity and health.

If I believe in the greatness of God and the majesty of God, if I know that God is so great and so big, and exists in all things that are good and in all of us, how can I fail to love myself? And if I love myself, how can I fail to love you?

Soul-Awareness

When I was living in Los Angeles, my assistant brought me to a church she thought I would enjoy. I walked in and saw this young pastor who was dressed like me, talking like me, sharing his story. When Pastor Touré Roberts spoke, I felt the energy and the connection moving through me and through the congregation. Everything he was saying, it was coming from his heart, and he was weaving the spiritual with the practical in a way that just made me want to take notes. Right away, I felt like I was in a welcoming space; it was the kind of feeling I hadn't had since Trinity in Chicago, and I knew right away that I'd be going back there. Every time I heard him speak, I left with things that I could work on. He became my pastor and my friend.

As he says, "Your soul is the deepest part of you, deeper than your mind, deeper than your spirit, deeper than your feelings. Your soul, that's the anchor of self."

PT, as he is known by our church family, is somebody I look to for inspiration because he approaches God from a spiritual place. He's not a preacher who operates from the idea that the church is right and the people living in the communities are wrong. That's something I appreciate about him.

PT is a human being with whom I feel so connected. We share

some of the same spaces and thoughts, and I've learned so much from him. He informs and inspires me, and there aren't many people I've met with whom I feel like I operate on such a parallel plane. We don't do the same things for work or for pleasure—he's a pastor who loves to ride motorcycles; I'm an artist who loves basketball. We didn't grow up together—he's from Watts, in Los Angeles—but we're only six months apart in age, and we just get each other. He was also raised by his mother, like me. I'll call him when I'm dealing with heavy things and when I'm rejoicing in hopeful things, or when I want him to pray with me on a relationship or a new play. We each bring a different aspect to the relationship, and we laugh and joke around, but we also speak to depth, and to wholeness, and to matters of the soul.

One thing we have in common is that we were raised by nurturing mothers and difficult fathers, and we have both walked a path to discover our own wholeness. Like Pastor Touré said, "The most important story in your life is a story you tell yourself." That's one of the things we talk about when we get together. How we define the world for ourselves, how to create that awareness around how we speak to ourselves. "All of us have a storyteller, and it's going to be in operation whether we're aware of it or not," he told me. "It's important for us to take control of that narrative."

Both PT and I have had to make peace with ourselves due to our relationships with our fathers. His dad was a Black Panther, a man who was very tough, had been through Vietnam. His definition of love was to prepare his son to live in this world by making him strong, by making him tough, too. His mother was nurturing; his father was all about preparation.

When he brought an achievement to his father, the response was, "How can you make it better?"

His father's toughness caused Pastor Touré's storyteller to constantly tell him, "You're not enough." That may not have been what his father meant to share, but that was the message he received. PT has shared that his father's approach created brokenness in his life that showed up as issues with authority. Anything that looked like authority, he was ready to fight. It took the process of knowing himself, self-awareness, to get to his wholeness.

When his father passed away, his dad's friends came around to tell him how proud his father was of him. "Your father was so proud of you," they kept saying. All the while, he was thinking that they just didn't know his father. By the end, he was in tears.

"After the last person came, I just broke down," he told me. "For me, wholeness is about being aware of the reality of your brokenness, understanding the damage of that brokenness and how that brokenness is causing you to show up in life." When you address those areas of brokenness with self-awareness, then you can show up as a whole person.

"Self-awareness is knowing yourself, knowing what you're doing and why you're doing it," he explains. "Self-awareness helps you to identify your areas of brokenness, which then helps you to get solutions and tools that will help you to re-center that."

He talks about two levels of awareness. There's self-awareness, and there's soul-awareness. As he describes it, "Self-awareness tells you where you are. Soul-awareness is deeper than that. Soul-awareness is the deepest part of you. The anchor of self is soul, and the soul has need. Being soul-aware is being tapped into what your soul needs. Soul-awareness is coming to a place where you know what your soul needs to be okay. It may be worship. It may be music."

For Pastor Touré, it may be reading scripture, praying, or meditating. It may be slowing down to connect with the longing of his soul. For you, it may be something else—to talk with a best friend, to be in the energy of a city, to sit by the stillness of a lake.

The important thing is to connect to the stillness of your soul because, as he put it, "Your soul is the most honest part of you."

"If you know your soul, if you're aware with your soul, you will interpret its cravings and longings and satisfy it appropriately," he explained, "instead of misdiagnosing your hunger and trying to satisfy your flesh, your humanity, your carnality when the real longing is happening in the deepest part of you, which is your soul."

This resonates with me because when I'm in my higher self, I'm about more than what my body is feeling. I'm more than my reactive emotions. Whether the emotion is jealousy or physical attraction to a woman, it's all energy. When I am aware of what my soul needs, my higher self can remind me that there may be a connection there, but that I don't have to act on it if the results won't be beneficial for me or that person. If it's impatience with another person, my higher self can tell me not to be reactive, but to meet people where they are, to understand that other people are going through things also. My higher self—that part of me that comes from my soul—is the most generous part of me.

Before Pastor Touré started his church, he was a successful businessman who would tell you that he was proud of his success. What he ultimately realized was that he did not have control over his urges.

"I was a promiscuous cat," he said. He wanted power over his body. He wanted power over his instincts and his urges. He wanted to be in control, and when he started going to church again, he discovered that he could go to church and still be himself. For him, it wasn't about being religious but about having spiritual power to be the highest version of himself.

"It was a new take on faith that drew me in as a young professional, as someone who didn't want to be confined," he said. Going to church gave him a new kind of freedom.

"You can still be successful, but you can be strong," he told me. "You can have strong willpower and not be moving in areas that are going to make you feel weak."

This revelation helped him, and the insights that emerged for him helped his friends, too. As he was sharing what he was learning, he found that people were compelled by these ideas, and the entrepreneur in him told him to create a framework through which more people could be exposed to the message. Without any background in church, he rented out a hotel and set it up so that he could reach more people; people who had a good heart, who wanted to be successful, who didn't want to be restricted, but wanted to live better and be better versions of themselves.

"It turned out to be much harder than I thought," he explained, "but that's how it started. I wanted to reach people like me."

From there, as he tells it, it just took off.

Pastor Touré has written books about wholeness, about awakening your purpose, and about balance. We talked about the balance you can experience when the soul is satisfied, when you're at rest. "I'm not talking about work-life balance," he said. "That's something different. That's new. I'm talking about balance as a place of rest and peace: your soul is content; you have an abundance mentality."

He reminded me that David said, "The Lord is my shepherd. I don't perceive lack." When you don't perceive anything as being lacking, from there, you just flow.

"No major accomplishment in my life happened from a place of rush and stress," he said. "It all happened from a place of rest. I don't care what it is. I've never stressed myself into success. I've rested myself into progress. And that's balance."

When you have balance, you're aware of what your soul needs and you satisfy the deepest part of yourself. In those moments, PT shared, "my wisdom is on another level because I don't have fear or this notion of I'm missing something to distract my energy. I don't have anxiety or worry stifling my creative ability, trying to remedy whatever it is I'm so worried about. My soul is at peace. So now, I can do what I do, and that is create. I'm created in the image of God, which means that I am a creator by design. The only thing that keeps me from creating freshly is when I'm distracted from the reality of my completeness."

As an artist, as a man, as a human being, this speaks to me in my soul. I'm constantly learning and inspired by PT and his wife, our copastor, Sarah Jakes Roberts. Their messages and friendship and support have blessed my life in unspeakable ways.

What I know is that thanks to my relationship with God, I can walk in my wholeness and my completeness. If you're communicating with the all-seeing, the all-powerful, omnipresent, omnipotent being, if you're communicating with that power first, you can overcome anything and be fruitful. You can connect with the purest and the greatest qualities that exist within you because you're connected to God.

A Light on My Path

I was living in a little two-bedroom place with my friend Rahsaan when I released my first album. I was twenty-one, and it was a nice little place in Hyde Park, and we were trying to make sure we could pay rent. The album wasn't successful, and I didn't know if I was going to get another opportunity. It was a scary place to be in. I went from knowing I had this album coming out to not being sure if I'd have another chance to record. I thought that when it was released, life was going to change, but life became more difficult when I released that album.

The dream didn't turn out like I thought it would. As I found myself in this place where I felt really challenged about where my life was going, I turned to my spirituality. Every day, I would read my Bible and pray, listening to God and seeking God. I was learning how to take those words and put them into practice. Even though I was in a space of doubt and darkness, I still kept saying the things that the Bible was teaching me, and it was reminding me that this wasn't just about this one album and one step. It was about this path that I was on, and this dream, and this purpose that I knew God had given me. It started with that one album, but it wasn't going to be finished with that one album.

If I wanted to get there, I had to stay on the path and continue to practice. Those actions of reading scripture, thinking about it, and applying it to where I was in my life gave me strength. I was reading other spiritual books that reinforced what I was learning from the Bible, and what I knew to be truth. I was making sure that my spirituality wasn't just a morning thing: it was something that I kept in my mental space and used throughout the day, and brought to mind when I was in those difficult situations.

As my practice has evolved, I continue to read my scriptures. This practice has helped me through so many moments. When I was dealing with memory issues after Covid, when I was worried about filming because it was harder to learn those lines, this was the practice that kept me steady. I kept reading my Bible scriptures. I continued my prayer. I just had to trust and be at that point, to be present.

I would get up in the mornings and say, "God, I know it's my purpose to do this. May this be for your higher good." And then I would take it with me through the day. I still do that. In time it was clear that while I put so much pressure on my first album, that first album didn't make or break. As long as you give your best and see where that takes you, you've got a whole journey to go.

When you let go of it just being on you, and being about you and what you're going to get out of it, when you think about what God wants you to be, and what He wants to receive from it, it takes the pressure off. You're giving it to the Creator, as if to say, "I'm going to do my part, God. You're going to do your part." I can trust in that. I do trust in that.

When you call an Uber, you trust that it's going to come and pick you up. If we can trust in that fact, if you can be confident in that, why wouldn't you be confident that when you call on God, He will be there? We should be even more confident because that's God. Reading scripture and connecting with God is part of finding success in life.

Everyone who is successful puts in the practice. When I was doing that play every day, even though I knew my lines, I still practiced on the way to the theater. I practice to win, to deliver, to be present. Steph Curry goes out there and shoots and shoots, practicing so that when he goes out on that court, he has that motion on recall. Even when he's being blocked, he can sink that ball. He doesn't have to think about keeping his elbow in when he's shooting. He's practiced that move so much that it has become part of his nature.

For me, practicing spirituality is part of my nature now. My practice allows me to be present, and in every situation, God is present with me. I know He is. That knowledge comes from me practicing, and communicating, and building that relationship with the Creator. It's that relationship and belief that has given me the foundation to take the step to recognize the God in me, no matter what happens.

That's something I have to remember when I'm in a meeting with a movie producer. I go in knowing I can lead movies, even though I haven't had leading roles in movies the way I thought I would. Does that stop me from acting? No. This is a path. It's an experience. When I come out of those meetings, I think to myself, *If this is the place I'm in, I'll be at this place. That's okay.*

One of my favorite pieces of scripture is Philippians 4:7–9. "And the peace of God, which transcends all understanding, will guard your hearts and your minds in Christ Jesus. Finally, brothers and sisters, whatever is true, whatever is noble, whatever is right, whatever is pure, whatever is lovely, whatever is admirable— if anything is excellent or praiseworthy—think about such things. Whatever you have learned or received or heard from me, or seen in me—put it into practice. And the God of peace will be with you."

Discovering that peace beyond understanding by putting God's word into practice is a lifelong journey. As an actor, I'm always going out for roles, and I don't get every part that I read for. If I audition and I know I didn't do it at the level I was supposed to, it irks me. It's going to stick with me. I've got to really work through that because I know that I didn't do it at my highest level.

If I don't bring my whole self to an audition, then I've cheated myself because I haven't given them a chance to see what I can really do. On set, when I'm filming something, I've got to give myself wholly, not knowing where my scene partner is at or how they might edit the scene we're filming. To let go and just be free in filming and acting takes a lot of trust, even if you're comfortable in front of the cameras. Whatever it is, I still have to give all of who I am.

If I audition and I went in there and I know I was centered and free and just did things in a way that was just present and I still don't get the role, I still feel some type of victory. You feel better when you give all of who you are. If you've really brought it, if you've tried at your highest level, then you can be proud, no matter what. Later, when I think back on it, I have to keep reminding myself that I was bringing the best I could. Knowing that is its own reward.

Sometimes, that part will go to another actor. When that happens, it's a natural feeling to experience jealousy, and to feel that rejection, because it can feel like they're saying, "No, you're not good enough," especially if I really wanted that role.

My mother reminds me that I trust in God, and I know that my purpose is to be doing what I'm doing. She's taught me that I can take those feelings of envy and turn them into something else. I'll send that person some light, say a prayer for them to go out and do great things, because when they got that role, it's because it was meant for them. When I get to my higher self, I can actually send that person good energy and love for that role and think to myself, *The next one is for me.*

That has helped me a great deal because holding onto the fact that I didn't get something, that someone else did, that they're out there playing in those films where I thought I could have done an excellent job—those feelings don't serve me in any way. When I release those emotions and turn them into something more elevated, into a prayer for someone else, I free myself. That puts me back into myself, who I am, what I want, what I can accomplish.

My peace beyond understanding comes from the relationship that I have with God. As I read scripture, and not just read it, but apply it, I see the power of God's words in connection with the power of my thoughts, my words, my actions, and my understanding. When I'm in my whole self, I can be around somebody that's doing more than me, selling more than me, more handsome than me, but I'm still happy with myself and feeling good because there isn't anything like that feeling of being my best self, of embodying the greatest part of me. With that in mind, I can appreciate and respect their greatness.

When you're in a place of gratitude, you can't really be jealous, you can't really be hateful to anybody, and you can't even really be angry. If you step into a moment of anger, when you bring God into it, when you say, "Thank you, God. I'm thankful that I'm here and that I'm breathing right now," you diffuse that anger; you erase that jealousy.

As human beings, we don't know what the future will look like. We invest our lives in things, and we don't know what that will mean for the future. We don't know how it will go. When you acknowledge God's great creations, when you trust what God created you for and for you to have, you can be present in your moments, present in your power, present in your whole self.

Finding Myself in the Stillness

I have been working on my spiritual practice for a long time, but it's only recently that I've come to appreciate the bounty that comes of finding stillness. For many years, my lifestyle was all about the work, all about going and moving and traveling from here to there. Beginning in 1996, almost thirty years ago, I've been on a plane every two or three weeks. I was always hustling, and the hustle became a way of life. My mantra was: *This is how you do it. This is how you get it. You've got to always be on the move.* That was my way to achieve my goals and reach success. I was always on the move. I was always on call and ready. If somebody popped up with something and they needed me to fly to New York for four hours, I did it. I got on the plane, flew in and performed, and got back on the plane the next morning.

Then the pandemic came upon us, and everything stopped. Before that, it was always "Let me work towards this because everybody's working" or "I'm missing out on something" or "I need to be working because this movie is in production" or "This person is releasing something new." During the pandemic, that mode of thinking was removed from our psyche. It wasn't part of the energy as a whole. I went to the raw core of what I needed in my life, what I loved in my life. I love building a relationship with God, and I used that time to be in conversation and listen and learn about God and with God.

During the early days of that era, I had space to find out what I really loved. I was reading God's Word, having time to be still, listening, meditating, praying, working out. Like it says in scripture, I had a peace beyond understanding. I felt connected to other people. I was not in competition. There was no ego.

In Philippians 2:1–4, it says, "Therefore if you have any encouragement from being united with Christ, if any comfort from his love, if any common sharing in the Spirit, if any tenderness and compassion, then make my joy complete by being like-minded, having the same love, being one in spirit and of one mind. Do nothing out of selfish ambition or vain conceit. Rather, in humility value others above yourselves, not looking to your own interests but each of you to the interests of the others." That's what I've been learning to apply in my life, via therapy and spirituality, so that I can live in my purpose.

Before the pandemic, people weren't as in tune with their spirits as they were when we were all going through that. We felt a certain thing together. We were all on this same wave, experiencing something together. That has a spirit in and of itself that you can't quantify or define all the way. It's the spirit of what a peace beyond understanding is. That's what the word of God means to me.

Having to be still during that period blessed me. My morning practices went from a rushed thirty minutes to a space where I could take as much time as I wanted. Not being on a schedule made me realize how important that time was for me, how important that morning practice of reading scripture and praying is for me. That was when I implemented meditation into my morning practice. Beforehand, I didn't have the time. During the pandemic, just being able to walk outside and look at the sun and see the trees made me happy and grateful. I felt gratitude at a deeper level; I felt my life in a new way. I felt my heartbeat in a new way.

I was able to connect with my family and friends, the people that I love in my life. In the past, rushing from one thing to the next, I never had time to talk because there was always a show or an event. When the world slowed, when I became still, I had time for deep and leisurely conversations. We got on a video call with my grandmother, and I saw her seeing her great-grandchildren, and my uncle, and it warmed my heart. I felt happy to be on and see my whole family. We don't have a big family, but we've got a loving family, and it's big enough. Making time for family is something that I didn't always prioritize before because I felt that all the grinding was helping me take care of the family. Back then, I didn't realize what I was missing. Now, I do.

Those days, I found myself doing the things that I just love. There was no outcome that I was seeking, no end. I was bouncing the basketball, working on drills, or shooting on the court, but it wasn't because I was training for a game, it was because I love it. I wasn't playing music to be hip to what's happening. I was just playing the music because I love music. I was watching old films instead of movies that I needed to watch for research, just watching for the love of it.

All of that showed me who I truly am. I learned that I revel in solitude. I love being able to have some time to myself, to be with myself and enjoy myself and not have to do anything but just be with me. It was a new experience to wholly occupy my time with things that I love to do and want to do. It was a renewal of who I am and what my soul needs. It allowed me to go forward with a focus on what I wanted to work on, what I wanted to create, what I wanted to practice.

What I was learning was how to be intentional. How to imbue my life with quality instead of quantity. To work out, to read, to listen to music, to enjoy a meal. It took me to the most simple things in life, how beautiful they are. I was able to build from there.

My vision is more focused and direct now. It's not all spread out or haphazard. That's how I love living, and I'm enjoying it. I still want to travel and see things and be able to be in New York, to go to Europe and do some work, to go to Ghana or Nigeria, and it's also a gift to love to come home.

Life can only be fully enjoyed and experienced when we truly understand what makes us the happiest. My thoughts about what it is to "make it"—those have been evolving, too. What I envision for myself, what I know God has for me here, the reasons that God has me here, I'm clear on that now. The whole thing is under God's umbrella of purpose.

We all have a higher purpose. Discovering yours is the true meaning of success.

One Day When the Glory Comes

"Welcome to the story we call victory
The comin' of the Lord, my eyes have seen the glory."

—"Glory," John Legend and Common

The ancestors are speaking. In "Glory," I can hear their voices in the words, in the rhythm, in that sound. When that song was released, it spoke to people. The world was being shaken by events that were occurring nationwide. Black people were being shot down in the street, and people were protesting more and more. That song touched people. It meant something to them. It was an anthem of our pain and of our hope, of our pride and our love for self and our love for God.

John Legend and I wrote "Glory" with Rhymefest for the film *Selma*, Ava DuVernay's portrayal of the people who marched the long miles from Montgomery to Selma in 1965 for the right to vote. It shows Dr. King's leadership and honors the contributions of the individuals whose efforts changed the world.

Dr. King was a true leader. He gathered the people around him, and everyone, from the teachers to the sanitation workers, committed themselves to the mission of justice, like the song says,

Shots, we on the ground, the camera panned up
King pointed to the mountain top and we ran up.

We don't know all their names, but that was their movement, these people who were working towards freedom and equality. It made me realize that life can't be just for you. God, children, family, community, nation, world—it's bigger than just you, and your role in it starts with you.

The film was produced by Oprah. There's a reverence and a respect and a deeply seated appreciation in it, and you can see it in all the research and love that went into it. James Bevel, my character, was a forward thinker who committed himself to the movement. As I was getting ready for the role, as I was learning to become that character, I was also learning for life. I was meditating on who it's good to be, who I might want to be, the footsteps I want to walk in.

So much happened in the world that coincided with the filming of that movie. On May 28, 2014, Maya Angelou, our hero, our teacher, our light, passed away. We were all on set together, Oprah and Ava and so many other people who loved Dr. Angelou. She meant so much to them, and she meant so much to me. I thought about everything I had learned from her and her warmth towards me. I remembered how blessed I was to be invited to her eightieth birthday party just a few years before. I freestyled for her that day, and I was so grateful to have been there, to rhyme for her, to do what I love for her, and for her to appreciate that.

One year before her passing, Dr. Angelou spoke with Oprah Winfrey on *Super Soul Sunday* and said, "I can do anything and do it well; any good thing, I can do it. That's why I am who I am, yes, because God loves me." She knew who she was, and she knew who we could be, and we loved her for it.

That day that she was called to transition, we all felt it. When we heard about her passing, we gathered on set and honored her with tears and with reverence, with joy, all of us Black people celebrating her and her life on this plane. She was a true queen, and she will never be lost to us.

Her influence shaped me and empowers me, and I can still hear her voice in my soul, telling me that she believes in me and that I can be better.

Dr. Angelou passed in the spring. By late summer, Michael Brown had been shot in Ferguson, and we were shown again that the past comes forward with us, that the pain repeats, that history is still being written. "Glory" was a song that illuminated the links between past and present and future. That song is about the events portrayed in the film, and it was also about what was playing out right in front of us. From Rosa Parks and the actions of our heroes, like Dr. King, from the march to Selma to Ferguson, it's all in there.

We were invited to perform "Glory" at the Grammy Awards and at the Oscars early the next year. It was my first time performing at the Grammys, and I was really nervous. First time, and we were going up after Beyoncé and closing the show.

That evening, I was caught up in the pressure. I was upset because the makeup artist was late, because I was using a new audio system and I wasn't used to it. I lashed out at my music director, and he grabbed me by the shoulders and gave me a little shake, as if to say, "Rash, what are you doing? Come back down to Earth."

That helped. The experience of this evening stayed with me in a positive way because I pledged to myself that moving forward, I was going to commit to doing all the things that would allow me to be present and be all of who I am in these big pressure moments. My knowledge of self has grown as a result. It has evolved. It really has become that peace within self, and discovering that peace beyond understanding is, for me, a great success. Wherever you are at now, whatever you are feeling, hold fast to your hopes for yourself because the rest of your life is a story that is as yet unwritten.

That evening, when we got onto the stage, I felt the spirituality in our performance because I knew that it was greater than us. It was God's music coming through in that song. I felt the presence of the ancestors, and because it wasn't about just us, it resonated more.

My soul has always yearned to be and grow closer to the most high. When the work that I do has a higher purpose and a greater meaning, it has the power to impact more people. That's where my soul is on the path.

When you offer love and care of self to your physical body, your emotional body, your spiritual body, you raise yourself up to a higher plane.

When you bring spirituality to what you do, when you do it with love, when you do it with purpose, you raise people's vibration and appreciation.

When you bring God into it, when you operate on a God level, when you recognize the higher purpose, the soul feels more fulfilled.

The qualities of love and joy and peace, kindness and patience, fruitfulness and abundance: these are your heavenly rights.

You are a child of God, created for happiness and to live life in wonder.

CONCLUSION

" There is nothing better for people than to be happy and to do good while they live. **"**

—Ecclesiastes 3:12

A Time to Plant

I was twenty-five when my daughter, Omoye, was born. That's the same age that she is as I write these words, which is strange to think about. When you're young, your parents look so old to you, even though they're young. Then you get older and become their age, which comes with a whole new realization of what they were going through as they were raising us up, and the cycle begins again.

I used to play John Coltrane to Omoye while she was in the womb. I would put the headphones on her mother's stomach and play music that I love to this baby we were having. I didn't know if she was a boy or a girl. I just wanted my child to receive this music.

Just seeing her come into the world was something. Along with this new, small person came all of my ideas of what I wished for, hoped for, and wanted for her. When she was born, I was still eating chicken. Her mother was a vegetarian. We had these conversations around what she would eat. Will she eat chicken, or won't she? We had our values, and we raised her to be aware of them. We would talk about her food, about her spirituality. Now I understand that it's about what she wants for herself.

I wanted to share my ideas with her and to make her aware of them, and I tried to give her the things that I thought would be helpful for her. Not all of it was. I remember one time I gave her some wheatgrass juice and we had to pull over and let her throw up. I felt like I was torturing my baby! To this day, she's traumatized by wheatgrass.

I have watched my daughter mature into a young woman who knows what the value of self-care is. She eats the food that she likes and that makes her feel good. She works out in ways that make her feel alive and strong. She was telling me how she was growing closer to God and building her faith, and she said, "You and mom told me these things, but I had to develop it for myself."

This was like music to my ears, the best music. That was like Stevie Wonder music to my ears, knowing that she was building her own relationship with God. It's something that she carries for herself. I planted seeds. It was up to her to water those seeds, to decide when it was time. She makes her own choices. To see her growing like this inspires me.

I remember talking with Omoye about centering practices when she was studying for the bar. We had conversations about the actions that help you get through, about how you've got to find those things that give you that grounding, whatever that looks like for you. As I told her, I can say what works for me. I can share my vision for myself. When it comes to your wellness, you get to develop your own vision.

The same goes for you. I want you to feel empowered by the ideas in this book. You don't need to do what I say. You can create your own practice that works for you. What doesn't call to you, leave where it is. Whatever information speaks to you is for you.

I saw that happen with my own mother. She observed what grew for me from the seeds I planted for myself, and she chose for herself that which spoke to her. My mother, who is a strong personality, who is a teacher and a boss, is aware of her food, eating a cleaner diet, taking spirulina and chlorella, working with Dr. Tracey, learning about the holistic practice along with the Western medicine. Now, when I'm visiting her, she'll say, "Let me give you this. I'm going to make your shake better. I'm going to put the spirulina in it." We learn from each other. Food is community and it is love, and that is really love when she's giving me the foods from her heart, and she's preparing it with healthier elements. It's good for all of us. Seeing her being conscious of what she's putting in her body, it shows me that we will never stop learning if we're open enough and if we're humble enough.

I can see her growing on a spiritual level, too. The way she talks about her relationship with God now has changed, as has her understanding of how powerful she is. When I was a child, I didn't understand that she was also young. Now I'm older than she was when we first listened to Reverend Wright's sermons at Trinity United Church of Christ, but I still feel young.

These are the cycles of life. We are born, we grow, we get older, and if we're lucky, we have our health, and we get to keep on learning. It's been a blessing to see my mother growing, to see myself growing, to see my daughter growing. None of us are perfect. We are all works in progress. We are all planting the seeds and watering the seeds. How we tend to our gardens of self is what influences the way we grow.

That's what I want for you. That's how I feel about this book. My teachers planted the seeds in me. I've planted those seeds in these pages. If you want these ideas to grow for you, you have to water the seeds for yourself.

A Time to Seek

Like it says in Ecclesiastes 3:1, "There is a time for everything, and a season for every activity under the heavens." This is your time. This is your season. Once you are on the path of loving yourself, you will be in tune with your own potential and your own power. Once you recognize that power, you can become a part of healing your community.

Remember, the power isn't a place you get to. The power comes from the process. Saying no to what is not good for you feels magnificent when you do it. So does saying yes to the positive. The discipline itself is power, and the results take you even higher.

I felt stronger when I went into that Thanksgiving dinner and said, "I'm not eating that." Hearing my cousins and uncles joking on me and still feeling that I was at peace with this choice because I was doing it for me—that gave me power. I knew they loved me and wanted the best for me, but only I could say what was truly best for me. At some point they started to say, "Wow, I understand this now, because you do seem happy, you do look good."

I had to recognize that within myself before they could see it in me.

I felt the power of moments where I said, "No, I'm not going to drink." I learned that I can be with friends, having a good time, playing board games, not drinking, enjoying myself, seeing who Rashid is without the alcohol. When I choose to have it, great. When I don't, that's also great.

It begins with a choice. From that choice, you know you're on a path, and you can keep pulling in those ideas that will benefit you. Maybe it starts with your morning routine. With drinking some green juice or doing a meditation. Maybe you read some scripture or some poetry. You can start walking, start working out, lift some weights, do a yoga class, whatever speaks to you.

You'll try things. Some will be tough. Some will feel good. When you stick with it, when you commit, you're really committing to you. No matter what's going on in the world, with your ambitions, with your family, with your creativity, you can rely on that commitment. You'll still be affected by what happens around you, but you'll also have a better way to deal with your struggles, to handle the challenges that arise. When those things do come, you won't crumble and fall. You'll have something that allows you to walk through it with some strength, with some understanding, with some compassion, with awareness.

The first section of this book is called "The Food." I've got a song by that title, too, with a line in it that goes, "I used to snap like a photo." I don't do that anymore. I'm measured. I'm thoughtful. That's the result of all these practices that I've committed to. When you've been taking care of you, if someone is giving you a hard time, when you're dealing with a lot, you might feel that pressure, but instead of instantly snapping or giving into emotional retaliation, you can rely on your higher self to help you through.

These ideas have delivered me to a place of great energy. I see the difference. I feel the difference. So do the people around me. Don't get me wrong, I have my moments with struggle, but overall, the path has brought me to a higher vibration, to my higher self, where I can really operate the way that I want to.

People in my community ask me, "What can I do?" The information in this book—that is one thing you can do. You can take care of yourself, and it will give you the energy to take care of others. If you've ever thought, *Why is Rashid smiling? Why does his skin look good? Why does his spirit seem like he in a good place?* It's because of these things that I've been doing, that I've been sharing with you.

We're all special, each and every one of us. Having those tools and resources to find the specialness in you will help you operate at that level in a consistent way. Every person that we mentioned in this book, each of them at some point found that thing within themselves. That's the place they're operating from. That's why they can be that light for me. Nobody does it without going through the difficult times and the challenges and the falls, the pains and the fears. Coltrane had to work through his issues to discover who he was spiritually, to create that music that inspires so many people. The fact that we're human doesn't take away from the fact that we have a higher self. It's all linked. We just have to reveal that to ourselves.

For me, I start to think about the vision that I have for myself and my goals and what I'm working towards. I need my energy, and I need to be awake and aware, and that's what my choices circle around. Physical strength. Emotional well-being. Mental health. Creative energy. Spiritual connection. These are what lead me. What leads you?

In Part 2, "The Body," I included a playlist of some of my favorite songs. One is a Black Sheep song called "The Choice Is Yours." It is yours. Nobody else's. Like Black Sheep says, "You can get with this, or you can get with that." What are you going to get with? What do you want for yourself? The choice is yours. Is it the right choice for you? Ask yourself, Does it feel like power? Does it feel like self-love? Does it feel like soul-awareness?

You've got the choice: it's yours to make. You can give yourself room to grow. You can open up space to have more in your life. If you want to be better, choose that.

Doing this type of work is the truest gift you can give to yourself.

SELF-REFLECTION
&
SOUL-AWARENESS

66 Just like hopes springing high,
Still I'll rise. 99

—Maya Angelou, "Still I Rise"

Hopes Springing High

And Then We Rise is a story about self-love. It's also a story about hope. Hope for self, for family, for community, and for future generations.

Earlier, I talked about the way Coltrane's *A Love Supreme*, his sublime, divine love letter to God, begins with "Acknowledgement." Acknowledgment is the source of all appreciation, all gratitude, all self-knowledge. That's where we are going to close this hopeful story: at a new beginning, with blue skies, on a clear morning, feeling self-empowered and ready to get into the majesty that is every single day.

Dr. Martin Luther King Jr. said that "Knowledge is a process of piling up facts; wisdom lies in their simplification." This book is a compilation of knowledge gathered over time by many people. In order for you to make it your own, you have to start from where you are, with a consideration of what you need.

Who are you? What brought you here? What are your hopes and dreams for yourself? Big questions, with layered answers that shift and change over time, but if we want to plant those seeds, we have to ready the soil. To truly acknowledge, you must have self-knowledge.

As you read these pages, what sections really spoke to you? What came to mind? What were you called to do? It may be related to a story that I told, or a stray phrase may have sparked something. Ask yourself, What ideas lit up for me, and how can I put them into action?

I've been thinking about how every one of my teachers, no matter what their field is, talks with me about self-reflection. It was from Dr. Tracey that I learned to take inventory of my body and what I needed so that I could approach my health care with more awareness. That's acknowledgment right there. Susan Shilling talked us through the HALT method, so we can root back into ourselves and figure out what our bodies need, so our minds can find calm. Pastor Touré's leadership calls us to listen closely and develop our soul-awareness, so we can fill those spaces with love. Yancy's approach to goal setting is rooted in who we are, how we want to show up in the world, what our innermost child—the one connected to a sense of adventure and fun—wants. All of these approaches are frameworks, mindsets, and exercises aimed at self-awareness and self-knowledge.

With all of that in mind, what comes next is a series of free-flowing questions that were created to inspire self-reflection. There aren't any right or wrong answers. There's only what you have experienced, what you hope for, what you want to bring into your life.

Every morning is another invitation to ask yourself the real questions. Like Yancy says, "Who do you want to be; how do you want to show up in the world?"

Reflecting on the Food

What drew you to this conversation about wellness and self-care? What does self-love feel like for you? What do you need in your life?

How can you start to give yourself what you need, in small ways or in bigger ways?

You don't need to go it alone on this journey. What kind of support would make you feel excited, inspired, ready? Nutritionists, emotional support groups, a group of friends you get together with to talk it all out . . . it's your journey. Who do you want as company along the way?

What has your relationship with food been throughout your life? Has it been calm and easeful? Tense and confusing? Something in the middle? Is nutrition something you think about regularly? Do you eat food that makes you feel good in your body?

Are you ready to eat more plants? At the grocery store, can you spend more time in the vegetable aisle, and fill your refrigerator with green vegetables, sweet squash, herbs, and fresh fruit before checking out the rest of the market? If you're a cook, can you get some cookbooks that call to you and try some new recipes? If you love restaurants, are there any vegetable-focused places that have opened that you've been wanting to try?

Who do you know whose food style really inspires you? Can you have a conversation with them? Eat with them? Hanging out with people whose choices magnetize us towards our higher selves is a powerful space to be in.

Honoring the Body

When is the last time you took a few moments to feel yourself? You can begin standing or you can lay down on the floor. Turn your head to the left and to the right. Stretch your arms above your head. Twist to the left and to the right. Where do you feel loose? Where do you feel tight? Where is your body at today? Is there an area that needs some warmth, some cooling, some love, some attention?

Where did your ideas about physical health and fitness come from? Are those healthy concepts to grow with? Are they perspectives you still want to hold onto? Or do you need a fresh take on your relationship with the human body?

What do you do to make yourself sweat? To feel limber? To feel energized? If you can't think of anything, this may be your moment to consider what activities you could launch into that will give you all of those feelings. Would you join a local group? Work with a professional? Get a live workout going with an app? Would you consider grabbing a bottle of water and heading out for a walk while you think about all of this?

Are there any parts of your body that you catch yourself complaining about or apologizing for? Do you have love and acceptance for all parts of you, even the ones people may have teased you about in the past, or the ones that catch your eye when you look in the mirror? When is the last time you gave your body thanks and gratitude for carrying you forward, for being the vessel for your soul, for doing what you ask it to do?

How has your sleep been lately? Is sleep something you prioritize, or does it always get pushed out of the way because there is so much to do in a day? What can you do to nurture your sense of rest, peace, and relaxation?

Nourishing the Mind

What would a well-balanced and fulfilling life look like to you? When you think of personal transformation, what might that involve? Imagine a flower turning towards the sun . . . what ways of being make you feel warm and connected? Can you write down one or two concrete steps that you can take to move yourself in that direction?

How connected are you to intellectual stimulation? How do you engage your curiosity? What gets you thinking? Do you travel? Do you explore your neighborhood? Do you try to do new things or create opportunities for yourself to grow?

Do you engage your artistic senses? Do you make space for art in your life? Listening closely to some music that you love, reading a book and letting the ideas sink in, going to see a play or to a museum . . . Painting, singing, playing an instrument, writing, crafting, designing . . . What art, literature, or music inspires you and leads you to your higher self?

What is your relationship to therapy? Do you have a space where you can talk with someone in a way that clarifies your sense of well-being and purpose?

Have you ever kept a journal? You can focus on goals and progress. You can make a list of recipes you'd like to try. Or you can just create your own diary of dreams . . .

Elevating the Soul

In this discussion of self-awareness, can you shift your attention to a deeper place and consider what Pastor Touré calls soul-awareness? What does your soul need to shine? Is it an action, a choice, a place, a person, a way of living? Can you give yourself that thing, that time, that energy, that space, that connection?

Where do you go to connect with your soul? Do you have

readings that you do, songs that you sing, a place of worship that you visit, a cathedral of nature you can go to in order to replenish spirit and connect with your higher self?

Do you offer thanks before you eat? Is grace something you grew up saying? Can you make space before meals to bring gratitude to the table? Saying thank you to God, to the people who made the food, to everybody who participated in growing the seeds, cultivating the land in order to make that meal possible for you changes the act of eating a meal into a spiritual experience.

Our souls are enriched by community connection. What does community mean to you? How does your community enrich your life? What do you do to support and uplift your community? What can you do? If community is something you want more of in your life, it works the other way, too: engagement with a community that is doing work that you respect is how you get to that place of connection.

We talked about the roots of spirit being breath. Can you take a deep breath in right now, and release it slowly, committing to nurture your spiritual side with your breath, with your words, with your intentions, with your actions?

What does your soul need to flourish and grow? What you wanted for yourself ten years ago, even last year, last month, might not be what you want for yourself today. The practice of self-reflection can help you illuminate your path and see yourself more clearly—who you used to be, who you are right now, and who you might become. In his liner notes to *A Love Supreme*, Coltrane wrote, "God breathes through us so completely . . . so gently we hardly feel it . . . yet, it is our everything." With everything you do, the spirit moves through you. Your higher self is part of you, waiting to be called upon.

As you connect with your higher self and choose your path forward, acknowledgment leads you to resolution. As resolution helps you create new commitments and put them into practice, you give yourself the chance to get to know the joys and pains of pursuance. As pursuance leads you down the path, as more and more evidence of lasting changes emerges, one day, you realize: you aren't just walking towards that promised land, that space of psalm.

You're already here.

NOTES

Part 1: The Food

1. "Black Food: Liberation, Food Justice, and Stewardship with Karen Washington and Bryant Terry," *Bioneers: Revolution from the Heart of Nature*, https://bioneers.org/black-food-liberation-food-justice-stewardship-karen-washington-bryant-terry/.

Part 3: The Mind

1. Laura Mehegan and G. Rainville, "2020 AARP Music and Brain Health Survey," AARP Research, June 29, 2020, https://doi.org/10.26419/res.00387.001.
2. David Haosen Xiang and Alisha Moon Yi, "A Look Back and a Path Forward: Poetry's Healing Power during the Pandemic," *The Journal of Medical Humanities* 41, no. 4 (2020): https://www.ncbi.nlm.nih.gov/pmc/articles/PMC7447694/
3. Andrew E. Budson, MD, "Why Is Music Good for the Brain," *Harvard Health Blog*, Harvard Medical School, October 7, 2020, https://www.health.harvard.edu/blog/why-is-music-good-for-the-brain-2020100721062.
4. "Black Americans and Alzheimer's," Alzheimer's Association, accessed September 11, 2023, https://www.alz.org/help-support/resources/black-americans-and-alzheimers.
5. "Black Americans and Alzheimer's," Alzheimer's Association.
6. "Minorities and Women Are at Greater Risk for Alzheimer's Disease," Centers for Disease Control and Prevention, last modified August 20, 2019, https://www.cdc.gov/aging/publications/features/Alz-Greater-Risk.html.

CONSIDER . . .

Reading the poem "Still I Rise" by Maya Angelou

Experiencing the album *A Love Supreme* by John Coltrane

Listening to the song "My Philosophy" by KRS-One

Getting a healthy start to your day with the cookbook *Eat Yourself Sexy* by Lauren Von Der Pool and by visiting www.laurenvonder pool.com

Bringing something from the cookbook *Vegan Soul Kitchen: Fresh, Healthy, and Creative African-American Cuisine* by Bryant Terry to your next family meal

Listening to this conversation between Karen Washington and Bryant Terry via bioneers.org, https://bioneers.org/black-food -liberation-food-justice-stewardship-karen-washington-bryant -terry

Reading *Eat to Live* by Elijah Muhammad

Reading the novel *Song of Solomon* by Toni Morrison

Working out with me and Yancy Berry on the YouTube show *Com + Well,* https://www.youtube.com/watch?v=HjzrYNXXsyI

Listening to the audio theater of *Bluebird Memories* by Common on Audible.com

Reading scripture via the Holy Bible

Reading the book *Balance: Positioning Yourself to Do All Things Well* by Touré Roberts, www.toureroberts.com

Seeing the film *Selma,* directed by Ava DuVernay

Listening to the song "Glory" by Common and John Legend

Experiencing the conversation between Oprah and Maya Angelou, *Super Soul Sunday,* May 12, 2013, https://www.youtube.com/watch?v=Irs5tJgokys

ABOUT THE AUTHOR

Common is an Oscar, Golden Globe, Emmy, and Grammy Award–winning music artist. He is an actor and producer, and has appeared in numerous critically acclaimed films, as well as in hit TV series. He is the author of *One Day It'll All Make Sense* and *Let Love Have the Last Word*, which were both *New York Times* bestsellers. He was raised in Chicago and currently resides in Brooklyn.

For additional content,
please follow the QR code below.